OPTIMAL TREATMENT FOR CHILDREN WITH AUTISM AND OTHER NEUROPSYCHIATRIC CONDITIONS

OPTIMAL TREATMENT FOR CHILDREN WITH AUTISM AND OTHER NEUROPSYCHIATRIC CONDITIONS

Dr. Jean-Ronel Corbier

iUniverse, Inc.
New York Lincoln Shanghai

OPTIMAL TREATMENT FOR CHILDREN WITH AUTISM AND OTHER NEUROPSYCHIATRIC CONDITIONS

iUniverse books may be ordered through booksellers or by contacting:

iUniverse
2021 Pine Lake Road, Suite 100
Lincoln, NE 68512
www.iuniverse.com
1-800-Authors (1-800-288-4677)

ISBN: 0-595-34892-0

Printed in the United States of America

Contents

ACKNOWLEDGMENTS

I thank God for helping me to complete this book. I would like to give a special thanks to my wife and son for their love, support, and assistance. This book is dedicated to all those who are involved in the struggle against autism.

PREFACE

"After reviewing all of the test results, I must conclude that your child has a condition called autism. This is a life long condition and there is no cure. Your child may never lead an independent life. You need to think about the possibility of institutionalization. I'm sorry." As you reflect back over the past three and a half years, you recall that your child was born healthy. You had high expectations for your baby. He began to develop normally and even seemed advanced. Then, between the first and second year of life, something strange happened. The baby stopped making progress. He lost the ability to speak and understand. The child became more and more withdrawn and seemed to be in his own little world. Then he began having annoying tantrums. There were long screaming fits for no apparent reason. At first you thought your child was experiencing the terrible twos a little early, but there was no sign of these tantrums decreasing not even after the third birthday. In fact, they got worse. The child who used to be such a good eater now has become very picky. There were also significant changes in mood and behavior that you noticed. Eye contact was lost. Little affection was demonstrated. There was an unusual fascination for certain objects and he had a tendency to line up or stack things endlessly. It is as if he seemed more interested in objects than people. He seemed to be such a strong willed child that you could not figure out what was bad behavior and what was due to a possible medical problem. He had repetitive movements. As you thought about the course of your child, it seemed undeniable that something significant had happened to him but what? How? Why?

After seeing the pediatrician several times and other specialists later on, the suspicion of autism is now finally being confirmed. Is that good or bad? At least now there is a diagnosis, but what does it all mean? Very little hope accompanies the diagnosis which only makes matters worse. You are shocked, and in denial. Then anger mixed with guilt and confusion sets in. The frantic search for answers begins, but as you learn more, you quickly become overwhelmed and are unsure about which direction to take. Multiple questions bombard your mind: What causes autism anyway? How treatable is the condition? Can it possibly be reversed or cured? What can be expected long-term? Which treatments of autism are safe, genuine and affordable? Then deeper questions emerge. Why was *my* child affected? Did I do something wrong?

The child's behavior worsens so you return to your doctor and desperately ask for some treatment. Drug therapy is immediately recommended. Although you have some concerns regarding the long-term safety of the drug prescribed, by this time you are almost at the end of your rope and feel the need for some type of treatment. You worry that you may need medication for yourself.

Unfortunately, many parents go through a scenario similar to the one depicted above. With more and more individuals being diagnosed with autism, it has become an important topic. The increasing prevalence of autism raises several questions such as why are more individuals being diagnosed with autism? Is the reported increased incidence due to better recognition of the disorder, or are there environmental triggers involved? What about vaccines? What does the latest research show? Is there any consensus on the cause and best treatment option for autism? Why is autism such a controversial field? In the midst of all of the controversies though, what can you do as a parent to make sure your child is receiving the best treatment options available with the right amount of support?

The purpose of this book is to introduce the reader to the importance of autistic spectrum disorders (ASD). Although a large focus of this book is on autism, this book concerns other neuropsychiatric disorders since many of the principles described in relation to autism also apply to other neuropsychiatric conditions. By *neuropsychiatric* I am referring to conditions that are either currently classified as neurological, psychiatric or that fall between both disciplines. In particular, I am focusing on neurobehavioral, cognitive and developmental disorders. I have specifically chosen to discuss autism because it is an all encompassing disorder that is intriguing and the most complex of the neuropsychiatric disorders. Children with autism, for instance, often have symptoms of attention-deficit hyperactivity disorder (ADHD), sensory processing disturbances, obsessive compulsive disorder (OCD), Tourette's syndrome, seizures, and a variety of metabolic-toxic-nutritional defects seen in several other neuropsychiatric disorders. This book provides a comprehensive look at autism using it as a framework to explicate other neuropsychiatric conditions. It also allows us to delve boldly into topics that are not usually addressed in books on autism. After an extensive examination of the nature of autism, we will discuss how it should be evaluated and treated. I end the book by describing what I consider the missing link in autism and other complex neuropsychiatric disorders. This part of the book is the most important and unique, putting things into the proper perspective. The missing link is explained by discussing a new model called the **RESTORATION** model. The **RESTORATION** model presents a fresh new look at autism and related disorders. It also provides a very encouraging treatment approach that is comprehensive and effective.

This book will specifically look at autism from all perspectives: neurobiological, neuropsychiatric, biomedical (nutritional, metabolic, gastrointestinal, immune and toxic), environmental, genetic, psychological, behavioral, philosophical and spiritual. In a broad sense, this book allows us to explore the mind, the brain, and human behavior through a detailed analysis of autism. To help the reader focus on the objectives of each chapter, I start with five poignant questions. The salient points are summarized at the end of each chapter. Owing to the use of some technical terms, a glossary is included at the end of the book. Perhaps most important, this book will provide hope for parents and caregivers of children with autism. True restoration of symptoms for autism and related conditions is believed possible if the right approach is used.

Jean-Ronel Corbier, MD

PART I

DEFINING AUTISM

1

HISTORICAL PERSPECTIVE

- What does the term autism mean?

- Where did the concept of autism originate?

- Is there an Austrian connection?

- Is there a relationship between autism and schizophrenia?

- Is autism a psychiatric disorder, emotional disturbance, a form of mental retardation, or is it something else?

Autism comes from the Greek word *auto* meaning self. The term *autism* was coined by psychiatrist Eugen Bleuler in 1912. Psychiatrists initially used the term autism to mean *escape from reality*. To say that someone was autistic was similar to saying that someone had escaped from reality, was out of touch with reality, or psychotic. It is this term, *autism*, that Leo Kanner used in 1943 to describe a group of 11 children (8 boys and 3 girls) with unique features. They had what he called "inborn autistic disturbances of affective contact". We now call this disorder autism.

Prior to the description of autism, as Kanner himself explains, these children were often diagnosed with childhood schizophrenia. Earlier, DeSanctis had introduced the concept of *dementia praecocissima*, and Heller spoke of *dementia infantalis* to describe early onset cases of schizophrenia. Theodore Heller was a special educator. He, like Kanner, was from Austria. Although the autistic children described by Leo Kanner had been confused with Heller's group, there were important distinctions that Kanner made in his original description:

1. In the early onset schizophrenia cases, there is at least two years of complete normal development followed by a gradual change in behavior. In Kanner's

3

original group these children seemed to have symptoms such as aloofness from the beginning.

2. Unlike the schizophrenic children, those with autism were able to establish and maintain purposeful and intelligent relation to objects that did not threaten to interfere with their aloneness. Kanner stated autistic children were "from the start anxiously and tensely impervious to people with whom for a long time they do not have any kind of direct affective contact....if dealing with another person becomes inevitable, then a temporary relationship is formed with that person's hand or foot as a definitely detached object but not with the person himself".

Autism, as originally described by Kanner, is a condition that has its onset during early childhood. The main characteristic is that of aloofness. Kanner used the term "autistic aloneness". The children described by Kanner appeared cut off from their surroundings. In addition, they had significant language and speech delay and were unable to properly use language as a means of communication. Finally, these children appeared to have a persistent need for sameness. They had repetitive movements called self-stimulatory behavior. They were prisoners of routine and structure. Kanner's particular contribution was the delineation of a special group of children with particular deficits that was unique and distinct from children with other disorders such as mental retardation, childhood schizophrenia, and other neuropsychiatric conditions. He explained that these children were not 'feebleminded' but instead "they are all unquestionably endowed with good cognitive potentialities...and have strikingly intelligent physiognomies". What that meant is that a child could have autism and be nonverbal without necessarily being mentally retarded or psychotic.

Who was Leo Kanner? He was a psychiatrist originally from Austria. He moved to the United States and eventually went to Johns Hopkins Medical Center where he practiced pediatric psychiatry. He is credited with having written the first pediatric psychiatry textbook. He also developed the first child psychiatry service in a United States hospital. Kanner was decidedly a prominent pediatric psychiatrist who was the chairman of child psychiatry at Johns Hopkins Medical Center for many years until his retirement in 1959. It is perhaps for this reason that many physicians have considered, and still consider, autism primarily as a psychiatric condition.

In 1944, one year after Kanner's original description of autism, a pediatrician by the name of Hans Asperger, also from Austria, described a set of children with symptoms similar to that of Leo Kanner's group. Asperger's group was much larger in number (over 400) than Kanner's group (of 11) but had symptoms that were very similar. Asperger's group was more diversified in their symptoms also. A large subset of children described by Asperger had a *later* onset of symptoms than those of Kanner. Many seemed to have normal or above normal intelligence, but had distinct oddities. Asperger used the term *autistic psychopathy*. It is interesting to note that both physicians used the term *autistic* independently in their original description. Both physicians were from Austria and they died within one year of each other (1980 and 1981 respectively).

In the next few decades autism, which was previously unknown and poorly understood, became associated with some strange theories. One such theory that was very popular was the psychogenic theory of autism proposed by another prominent individual, a third Austrian figure, Bruno Bettelheim. Bettelheim was a developmental psychologist/psychotherapist who had a special interest in childhood developmental disorders. He became famous for his work with emotionally disturbed children. From 1944-1973 he was the director of the University of Chicago Sonia Shankman Orthogenic School for severely troubled children. He also taught psychology at the University of Chicago. He felt that autism was the result of parents, mothers in particular, who were cold and distant toward their infant. The psychopathology of the mothers eventually translated into a cold, aloof, autistic child due to poor maternal-infant bonding. It followed that the proper treatment for such a condition would entail removing these children from their home environment and placing them in a more loving, warm and nurturing milieu. This is how the notion of the *refrigerator mother* developed. Bettelheim wrote: "all my life I have been working with children whose lives have been destroyed because their mother's hated them." Mother's of children with autism were described as being cold and unable to form a warm loving bond with their infants. Imagine that after carrying your baby for 9 months and having high expectations for the child, you are informed that your baby is abnormal and has a dreadful condition called autism. Then, before you have a chance to regroup, you are blamed for it and your child is taken away from you! Bettelheim's theory was actually a prevalent and accepted theory for many years.

Apart from the fact that Bettelheim suffered from depression and died by committing suicide in 1990, it has been discovered that many of his stated academic accomplishments were fabricated. Although in his lifetime he was well respected and viewed as brilliant for his work at the Orthogenic School in Chicago, it was later discovered that he was a cruel tyrant. It is interesting to note that Bettelheim's theory was accepted not only by psychiatrists, but scientists and many others. Looking at the history of autism, we ought not to make the same mistake today. Autism must be understood properly to prevent suffering of the children and their families.

Dr. Bernard Rimland in 1964 wrote a book (Infantile autism: The syndrome and its implications for a neuronal theory of behavior) that challenged Bettelheim's psychogenic theory, suggesting that autism was instead a biologically-based disorder. In 1977 Dr. Susan Folstein and Dr. Michael Rutter published the first twin study of autism suggesting a genetic link. Further research confirmed that autism is indeed a biological disorder. Now that autism is known to be a biological disorder, the next question is what causes this biological disorder? As we will see later on in this book, that is a complex question but it can be answered accurately.

Key Points

- Leo Kanner, a child psychiatrist originally from Austria, was the first person to describe autism.

- Hans Asperger, also an Austrian physician, independently described autism at approximately the same time. He looked at a broader spectrum of presentation in children with autism and looked at a much larger group.

- Early theories of autism hovered around a psychological or psychiatric etiology.

- Bruno Bettelheim introduced the psychogenic theory of autism, blaming cold parenting for the condition. This theory was dismantled in large part by Dr. Bernard Rimland.

- Although psychological and psychiatric disturbances are present, autism is now viewed as a biologically-based disorder.

2

FULL SPECTRUM OF AUTISTIC DISORDERS

- What exactly is autism?

- What is the difference between Autism, Asperger syndrome, PDD and ASD?

- Is there any relationship between autism, OCD, ADHD and Tourette's syndrome?

- What conditions mimic autism?

- How many types of autism are there?

What exactly is autism? Autism is a disorder that starts in early childhood and is characterized by deficits in the following core areas:

1. Communication

2. Social interaction

3. Behavior

At its worst, children with autism are seemingly cut off from their environment. They appear to be *in their own little world.* They seem unable to speak or comprehend language. They do not interact appropriately with other people and often have episodes of severe and lengthy behavioral outbursts. They also have self-stimulatory movements which may include rocking, hand flapping, walking on their toes or looking at objects from the corner of their eyes. These behaviors may occur for prolonged periods of time.

With milder cases, an individual may be verbal and even speak very clearly, but there may be problems with intonation (monotone voice) and spontaneous, conversational language. Behavioral problems in the milder cases may be expressed mostly in times of stress. These individuals may interact socially, but still lack social cues. Things may be taken very literally. Most individuals with autism appear normal physically. Today, we find that children with autism have a greater range of affection that still encompasses the diagnosis of autism.

Autism, PDD and ASD

Autistic symptoms can be seen in several disorders. This has led to the psychiatric umbrella term of *Pervasive Developmental Disorders* or (PDD). According to the Diagnostic and Statistical Manual of Mental Disorders Fourth Edition (DSM-IV), there are 5 conditions that fall under this rubric:

PERVASIVE DEVELOPMENTAL DISORDERS (PDD)

- Autism

- Asperger's Disorder

- Childhood Disintegrative Disorder

- Rett's Disorder (Rett syndrome)

- Pervasive Disorder Not Otherwise Specified (PDD-NOS)

Asperger syndrome

Asperger syndrome is a condition initially described by Hans Asperger in 1944, but he actually used the term *autistic psychopathy*. Because of the possible confusion of the term *psychopathy* with that of *sociopathy* which is very different, Lorna Wing, researcher from England wrote a paper in 1981 entitled: Asperger syndrome: A clinical account in which she suggested that the name be switched from *autistic psychopathy* to *Asperger syndrome*. There are arguments concerning whether Asperger syndrome represents a form of high functioning autism or if it is a separate condition. A main feature of this syndrome is that it appears to be inherited. Occasionally there is an undiagnosed 'odd family member'. It is much more common in males. Unlike Kanner's original description, many children with this condition have very good verbal skills from a very early age, although there are various aspects of language that may be impaired. The voice may be monotone, and there may be areas of interest that are significantly restricted. An example would be fascination with a certain class of insects, or a particular fascination with astronomy. There tends to be significant clumsiness. A good visual image of a child with Asperger syndrome is a small child that can name every bone in the body or can name various stars and galaxies but cannot tie his shoelaces. Many children with Asperger syndrome have normal or above normal intelligence. Mood and anxiety disorders such as obsessive compulsive disorder are common in these children. Many have significant *mind-blindness* and are very literal and concrete (see Chapter 6). Why do individuals with Asperger syndrome acquire their symptoms late instead of from the start? Do they have an underlying disorder or are they merely odd? Or was what Hans Asperger believed true, that these children had a 'psychopathic' personality trait? Perhaps there is a combination of inherited personality trait with a relatively mild underlying disorder (that is relative to Kanner's definition of autism).

Childhood disintegrative disorder (CDD)

Another category of children with autistic symptoms is that of Childhood Disintegrative Disorder (CDD). It is also called Heller's syndrome, dementia infantalis, or disintegrative psychosis. Unlike children with autism, these children, usually boys, do not develop their symptoms until after several years of previous normal development. Usually symptoms start between 2 to 4 years of age, but may not start until 9. This condition is thought to be much rarer than Kanner's autism, and the prognosis is worse. This enigmatic condition is very interesting from an analytical standpoint for several reasons. It is presumed to be due to some neurologic dysfunction since it is associated with seizures, and there is a definite regression in a variety of areas including bowel and bladder control. Why is the onset of this condition so late? Why does it present later than autism? Why is it much more prevalent in males? Why is it so rare, 1.7 per 100,000? Why is the outcome worse than autism? How does one explain the lack of objective findings in many cases? These questions are addressed later on in the chapter.

Rett's syndrome

In the PDD group, the only disorder to occur almost exclusively in females and to have a known gene defect is Rett's syndrome. It is caused by a defect in the MECP2 gene on the long arm of the X chromosome—Xq28. Males can get the syndrome, but it is lethal in the fetus. Since the chromosomal abnormality occurs on the X chromosome and females have two X chromosomes, they are protected and do not experience fetal death when they are affected. In this condition, a female infant who was previously normal, after 6–18 months of age starts to develop microcephaly. Eventually, the child develops other cognitive defects and finally starts appearing autistic, losing acquired speech. There is a characteristic hand-ringing that develops, representing loss of purposeful use of their hands. Severe seizures may develop as well as hyperventilation and other breathing abnormalities. All symptoms are progressive, making this a neurodegenerative condition, although children with this condition often reach adulthood.

There are several lessons to learn from this particular condition. First, although it is listed in the PDD category, it is a specific condition with a known etiology, clinical outcome, and pathogenesis. Therefore, any female child diagnosed with autism (or cerebral palsy) who is microcephalic should be worked up for Rett's syndrome, especially if there is accompanying mental retardation. Second, although most autistic disorders have a male predominance, Rett's syndrome occurs almost exclusively in females for the reasons explained above. Third, although children with Rett syndrome appear to have autistic symptoms, a specific underlying genetic condition has been identified. This suggests that in a subset of individuals with autism, a specific gene abnormality may result in their autistic symptomatology.

Pervasive developmental disorder not otherwise specified (PDD-NOS)

Finally, there is a group of children with autistic features that do not fit in any group. Symptoms may start very early with some degree of mental retardation, which would make both Asperger syndrome and childhood disintegrative disorder unlikely. Because some autistic features may be very mild or absent, criteria for autism may not be clearly met. This group, which may be the largest, is set aside and placed into the category of pervasive disorder not otherwise specified (PDD-NOS). With PDD, although several disorders are grouped into one category in the psychiatric manual (DSM-IV), the underlying conditions may be quite different. Autistic symptoms can vary from relatively mild to severe making the more recent term *autistic spectrum disorders* (ASD) a more appropriate one. In the remainder of this book I will use the term autistic spectrum disorders interchangeably with autism.

CURRENT DIAGNOSTIC TOOLS

There are a variety of diagnostic and screening tools available to identify children with autism that rely on rating scales and observation. Some common examples include: ADOS (Autism Diagnostic Observation Schedule), ADI-R (Autism Diagnostic Interview-Revised), CARS (Childhood Autism Rating Scale), GARS (Gilliam Autism Rating Scale) and CHAT (Checklist for Autism in Toddlers). The main purpose of these standardized tests is to identify behavior, social, and cognitive characteristics that are consistent with autism and eliminate those that are consistent with other problems such as mental retardation or other cognitive abnormalities. Many of these rating systems also allow categorization of autism based on severity. Some of the screening tools such as CHAT allow detection of symptoms as early as infancy. Lack of pointing as a form of shared attention (called protodeclarative pointing), has been found to be one of the earliest indicators of autism. Another early sign is lack of pretend play.

Limitations of current diagnostic tools

What are the limitations of current diagnostic systems? A diagnosis of autism using the above diagnostic tools is based on a set of criteria (often psychiatric, e.g. DSM criteria) based only on a child's behavior, communication, and social impairments deemed severe enough to result in functional limitations. When the label of autism is applied, educators, psychologists, lay individuals and clinicians may view the child in a manner that does not necessarily reflect the wide range of underlying problems that may be present. It is important, in my opinion, to incorporate information regarding the suspected etiology of the disorder and identify any biological problems present (such as seizures or an underlying brain defect) in developing the diagnosis of autism. Why is this essential? If an etiology is considered in making the diagnosis, then treatment protocols can be individualized and targeted based on the suspected etiology. Prognostic issues can also be discussed with greater accuracy and confidence.

Another limitation in the current diagnostic scheme is that rating scales can be very nebulous at one end of the scale. Imagine a child who does not quite qualify according to the rating system. Let's say that the child is one point shy of qualifying for the diagnosis. That child, according to a given rating scale may not have autism, although in reality, the underlying pathology may be similar to someone who has more severe symptoms that do qualify him for a diagnosis of autism. At best, the evaluation process should be aimed at ruling in or ruling out the presence of autistic spectrum disorder. The level of severity can then be addressed. There should be no borderline cases. Mild autism should still be considered autism since such an individual, under stress or with certain triggers may manifest much more severe symptoms.

There are many conditions that may superficially mimic autism but may have a completely different set of etiologies (such as particular structural brain disorders or a psychogenic disturbance) and require a different treatment approach. For example, a child that is mute due to a structural brain defect who also happens to be shy may superficially appear autistic. A careful examination may reveal that the child has great receptive language abilities, good social skills, and has no sensory deficits or other disturbances commonly encountered with autism. Such a child should clearly not be diagnosed with autism. I do not find the term PDD-NOS useful. In my practice, children that present with some autistic traits but in which there is no clear genetic diathesis, we have chosen to use the term *autistic equivalent.* Clearly, there are many disorders and there are many personality traits that can include some autistic features without causing functional impairment. By properly including the 'borderline' cases into the category of autism, many individuals may be caught who would otherwise fall through the cracks in the current diagnostic scheme. Without a proper diagnosis these individuals could encounter problems in school and other settings that would not be able to be explained. This would lead to frustration on the part of the family, child, and society.

Autism can present in a variety of forms and is therefore not one disorder but a syndrome caused by various processes. Below are 5 simulated patient cases with autistic symptomatology that highlight the range of presentations that can be encountered:

Case 1

Raymond is a 35 year old male who lives with his aunt and uncle. He has a job and is semi-independent, but is frequently shadowed by his aunt or uncle because of his problems with social interaction. Raymond is well-mannered and well groomed. He is nice, but socially inept. It is easy for individuals to take advantage of him. He has odd mannerisms and likes to rock back and forth, especially if he is nervous or stressed. He also tends to walk on his toes, but can walk flat footed if reminded. He does not like to wear a tie and sometimes his clothes do not match, but he is open to suggestions regarding his dress. He seems to have a photographic memory and can tell you the day of the week for any date that you give him over the next five years. His sense of direction is excellent, although at the same time he does not comprehend some simple things. He can add any number in his head, but cannot solve simple practical problems.

Retrospectively, as in infant, Raymond had mild delays in developmental milestones, especially language. Compared to his older siblings his speech was delayed. This was the first clue that something was wrong. From early childhood, he was found to be very routine-oriented. He thrived in a structured environment, but would have prolonged tantrums if his routine changed even slightly. Some of the tantrums seemed to come out of the blue with prolonged screaming fits. As a child, Raymond liked to line up and stacks objects. He had an unusual fascination for certain objects, particularly ones with wheels and spinning objects. Raymond had a tendency to wake up very early, like clockwork, no matter when he went to bed. There seemed to be a routine, order, and symmetry with everything. The most predictable way to cause a tantrum or meltdown would be to alter his things. His language development was slow, but eventually improved. However, his speech remained laconic and very literal. Eye contact is still poor, but improved. Raymond has a cousin who was diagnosed with Asperger's syndrome. For many people who know Raymond superficially, they view him as a nice guy who has some oddities and lack of social cues.

Case 2

Joanne is now 15 years old. Her main problem at presentation was that of recurrent seizures and speech delay. She also has cognitive delays. The parents' earliest memories are of a very fussy and agitated infant. She was hard to console. All of her developmental milestones were delayed. She initially seemed floppy then became stiff in the lower extremities. As a toddler, she always walked on her toes. Reminding her to walk flat footed did no good since she was physically unable to do so. She started having staring spells with altered responsiveness at the age of 4, and her first grand mal seizure at the age of 9. She has a least 3 to 4 grand mal seizures per month. She is very clumsy and is in special education classes. She has all of the classical signs of autism and the neurological problems mentioned above. Her neurologist has diagnosed her with cerebral palsy. Her speech is significantly delayed. There are times when she seems lucid and says some words clearly that you did not think she knew. But at other times she seems almost mute, usually the days following an exacerbation of her seizures.

In addition to cognitive delays, Joanne has clear evidence of a neurological disorder. She has a cousin with a rare metabolic disorder and a sibling who also has speech delay. She has been diagnosed with cerebral palsy with autistic tendencies. The neurologist has suggested that Joanne may have a neurometabolic disorder presenting with autistic features and cerebral palsy. Further studies have been recommended.

Case 3

David is now an 8 year old male who is well adjusted, mainstreamed in a regular 3rd grade class, and doing well. No one who does not know David's past history would guess that David had full fledged autism when he was younger. He had been diagnosed independently by 2 professionals when he was age 3, although there were suspicions previously. He started having recurrent ear infections when he was only 4 months of age and was placed on multiple rounds of broad spectrum antibiotics. He was also congested and had very loose stools. He had severe gastroesophageal reflux and was placed on a variety of different formulas as an infant. Despite being sickly, he did well socially and linguistically, until between 15 and 18 months of age. Then there was an insidious, but definite change. David became withdrawn, and was no longer an affectionate child. He often looked dazed as if in another world. Sometimes he acted as if he were deaf, although subsequent hearing tests were normal. He frequently seemed overwhelmed by certain sounds and crowded situations. He became extremely aggressive, hyperactive, and inattentive. Overall, he was difficult to deal with. He stopped eating most foods, except for fries and chicken nuggets, and seemed to crave cheese and wheat food products. Things started changing when David's parents saw a DAN physician who recommended removing gluten and casein from his diet. The parents decided to undergo a whole lifestyle change. Since both parents and another sibling also have autoimmune disorders and have themselves had recurrent infections, the entire family decided to eat healthy. This has made a remarkable difference in everyone's health.

Although David initially required intensive behavioral, speech, occupational, sensory integration, and auditory integration therapies, he seems to have overcome his autism. He is now happier, pleasant and turns out to be a very bright, sensitive, affectionate child. Though he has a few problems, his last psychological tests show that he no longer fits within the autistic spectrum.

Case 4

Jeanne and Jane are 15 year old identical twins. Double trouble! Both have been diagnosed with Asperger's syndrome. The diagnosis was made at the age of 12 years. Previously there was a laundry list of diagnoses given by several specialists including: ADHD, OCD, Tourette's syndrome, chronic depression, chronic mood disorder, bipolar disorder, adjustment disorder, oppositional defiant disorder and post-traumatic disorder. The last clinician who evaluated the girls was specialized in the evaluation and treatment of ASD/Asperger's Syndrome and explained why the prior specialists failed to come up with the diagnosis of Asperger's syndrome. The clinician explained to the parents that because the girls were very advanced linguistically when they were very young, it would have made such a diagnosis difficult. The parents had also noted that the girls were reading well with good pronunciation before the age of 4. The parents actually were convinced that the girls were geniuses and had high hopes for them. But then, they started to develop signs of hyperactivity, mood changes, and later severe obsessive compulsive behavior. One of the girls, Jane, became so suicidal that she had to be hospitalized in a psychiatric ward for several days. Academically, the girls were straight A students, and were found to have very high IQs. They did, however, have significant social interaction difficulties. They lacked tack and got in trouble with their peers because of their comments. When asked how a dress looked by one of her friends, Jane responded that it was the ugliest dress that she had seen. She could not understand why that made her friend upset. She was just telling the truth. Both girls were often melancholic and had severe mood swings that almost became unbearable when they entered puberty. Interestingly, there was a long standing history of mood and anxiety disorder on the maternal side of the family. The girl's father was phlegmatic with little intonation in his voice. He was not very outgoing, but compared to the other males in his family he was apparently the most interactive and outgoing.

Case 5

The final individual, Giovanni, is an adult who has never actually been diagnosed with anything. At one point when he was younger, he was taken to a psychologist because he had significant problems with hyperactivity, attention span, and some school difficulties. He did interact socially but was very shy and never initiated a conversation, though he would respond appropriately. He did better with one-on-one interactions than with groups. He did have some autistic symptoms that were mild and apparently spontaneously resolved. Giovanni, who is now a successful chemical engineer, believes that his success can be attributed to a life of good nutrition, proper family/social/spiritual support, and normal brain development. Although Giovanni does not have any family history of autism, there is a family history of ADHD, tic disorder, and one individual with chronic illness as a child. That individual which had chronic illness suffered from severe asthma, allergies, and upper respiratory infections, but was unusually bright with excellent grades in school. There were mild social interaction difficulties and the individual was moody.

The outcome, underlying abnormalities and treatment options vary significantly in each of the cases presented above. These cases demonstrate the need for a more effective way to diagnosis ASD. I propose using a system of categories to determine not only if an individual has autism, but the treatment option which would be most beneficial. The importance of evaluating autism based on pre-determined categories can maximize the likelihood of proper treatment options for patients based upon the particular category that applies to them. Instead of diagnosing an individual with "autism" or ASD, one might instead diagnose an individual with a specific *type* of autism representing a category applicable to their particular clinical condition.

Parameters that should be considered when a formal diagnosis of autism is made include:

- Time of onset of autistic symptoms. A child who clearly had symptoms from early infancy or birth is different from one who did not show any signs until 2 ½ years of age or more. It should be noted, however, that many children who do not have autistic symptoms until later on, may still have other abnormalities such as reflux, recurrent infections or milk intolerance during infancy. These children may be susceptible even in their pre-symptomatic state.

- Systemic involvement. For instance, a child who only has communication, behavioral, and social deficits is different from a child who has autism in addition to gastrointestinal, immune, or additional neurological disturbances.

- Presence of regressive symptoms. Some children may have acquired language and social skills normally before regressing into autism. Children with regressive symptoms and children with late onset autism may have a toxic, metabolic, infectious, or iatrogenic cause for the development of autism. Of course these children must have a genetic susceptibility. SEIZURES SHOULD ALWAYS BE CONSIDERED IN THESE CASES!

Types of autism:

One way to differentiate between the types of autism is the onset of symptoms. Some children have symptoms from birth (primary autism) and others develop symptoms after the age of one or two years (acquired autism). This latter group can be labeled as having regressive autism, secondary autism, or acquired autism.

- Primary or congenital autism

    This group may or may not present with mental retardation, although mental retardation is more likely in this group. Kanner's original description of autism was likely comprised of individuals in this group. These children may have a congenital defect that may be present even before birth. These are the children who may have the most difficulty with speech. There is no obvious regression of symptoms. This group is best labeled as having **primary** or **congenital autism.** These children may have some neurometabolic, structural brain defect, or specific genetic abnormality. The goal of investigation in this group is to try to identify a very specific disorder that caused their symptoms, and to treat it as specifically as possible to prevent further damage.

- Secondary or acquired autism

    Other children with autism seem to have acquired or regressive symptoms usually between 1 ½ to 2 ½ years of age. Many were initially noted to have normal eye contact, social, and language development. Then abruptly or insidiously, noticeable changes occur. The child starts behaving as if he/she is deaf, loses appropriate eye contact, and may no longer be affectionate. The child may be in a *fog* state several minutes or hours at a time. Interestingly, in some of these children there are periods of intermittent lucidity. These periods of lucidity may appear haphazardly, during or following an infection, during particular periods of the day, or at other times. These episodes may occur frequently enough to let the parents suspect that there is a potentially normal child that is trapped inside a complex matrix that inhibits proper social inter-action, communication, and behavior.

With these children who were developing normally or in many cases were clearly advanced, one has a sense that there has been a specific insult to the brain and body that has caused the child to regress. These children have fluctuations in their symptoms. Some of these children at times may appear normal, and at other times the full characteristics of autism are manifested. The increased cases of autism seen in recent years have in large part reflected children in this category. This group is best labeled as having **acquired** or **secondary autism.** In this group, many individuals may have normal (or above normal) intelligence. There may be reports of an association with heavy metal toxins, immune disturbances, multiple food allergy/sensitivities, and gastrointestinal disturbances. I speculate that children with childhood disintegrative disorder really fall in this category. They may have a particular gene defect that may cause them to succumb to an environmental trigger. The trigger can be something quite rare, such as an unusual viral infection, or something common that most individuals do not have susceptibility for. Autoimmune disturbances may also be present in these individuals.

Another way to categorize autism is to look at predominant biological defects that may be present. Based on this model it is possible to come up with a system that takes into consideration the various systemic dysfunctions seen in autism. Such a tool would allow a clinician not only to identify potential areas of concern but this would also help the clinician focus on an appropriate treatment protocol. Having a *biological/biochemical autism rating system* or **BARS** would also sensitize families to the areas of dysfunction present.

Examples of categories emphasizing biological dysfunction would include:

- Gastrointestinal-dominant autism (severe primary gastrointestinal abnormalities)

  These autistic children may have chronic loose stools, gastroesophageal reflux, infant formula intolerance, fussiness during infancy, leaky gut syndrome, recurrent yeast infections, and evidence of chronic malabsorption. They may have significant behavioral problems. These children may do very well with such interventions as probiotic and antifungal treatment, specific carbohydrate diet, secretin therapy, and a gluten/casein-free diet. In these cases correction of gastrointestinal abnormalities may be associated with dramatic improvement of overall symptoms. These children can also have an immune disturbance that contributes to the gastrointestinal problem.

• Immune-dominant autism (severe primary immune abnormalities)

In this group of children with autism there is evidence of immunological problems manifested by recurrent respiratory and ear infections beyond what is seen in other children with or without autism. There may be a strong family history of autoimmune disturbance. Side effects from vaccines/Thimerosal are more likely in this group. Secondary gastrointestinal disturbances may become evident due to overuse of broad spectrum antibiotics and yeast overgrowth. Nutritional interventions, with an aim of boosting immune function, may prove useful (i.e. intravenous glutathione, colostrum, glyconutrients, and other strong antioxidants). Intravenous immunoglobulin may especially be helpful for refractory seizures and neuroautoimmune dysfunction.

• Neurological-dominant autism (severe neurological problems, refractory seizures)

In this group there may be cognitive delays, frequent seizures, muscle tone abnormalities, significant tic disorders, and other evidence of neurological dysfunction more pronounced than in other groups. This is the group that should always have an EEG (possibly a 24-hour if necessary), neuroimaging (MRI), as well as a very comprehensive neurometabolic evaluation looking for specific inborn errors of metabolism. Genetic testing should be considered. Anti-epileptic therapy may prove very useful if seizures are present. The challenge in this group is to identify the specific underlying problem and to treat specifically.

• Pseudoautism

Pseudoautism is a term that has been applied to a specific condition where a person manifests autistic symptoms caused by lesions in the posterior parietal cortex bilaterally. These children often have an associated disorder of mood and affect. When the mood disorder is treated, communication usually improves markedly.

There are a variety of other conditions that may present with autistic symptoms. The symptoms may be transient or chronic. These conditions may resolve with time without the usual therapies for autism. There are some children with a diagnosis of ASD that fit in this category whose problem will disappear independent of any treatments or therapies used. Children in this category would include children that have been severely neglected or abused early in their life. These children may develop signs and symptoms similar to autism. Although they may have a lot of 'catching up' to do, if placed in a caring and loving home their symptoms may reverse. These children may receive speech and other therapies, but the best intervention for them is being placed in a supportive environment. Assuming their brain is healthy, these individuals can normalize. This is not to be confused with Bettelheim's erroneous psychogenic theory. He blamed normal mothers for their child's autism. In this situation, if there is a problem such as neglect, abuse, or social isolation, the symptoms may resolve if the environment changes.

Other conditions that fit into this category would be children with auditory abnormalities and chronic ear infections causing partial hearing deficits. Such a child can appear to have autistic symptoms. Clearing up the ear infections and correcting the hearing loss, can cause the 'autistic symptoms' to disappear.

CONDITIONS THAT MAY MIMIC AUTISM

- Elective mutism

- Childhood schizophrenia

- Congenital deafness

- Mental retardation

- Congenital ocular/cerebral visual impairment

- Retrolental fibroplasias

- Septo-optic dysplasia

- Pseudoautism

- Epilepsy-related syndromes

  - Landau-Kleffner Syndrome (LKS)—acquired aphasia (language/speech disturbance) in association with seizure discharges in the temporal/parietal regions.

  - Epilepsy with continuous spike-wave discharges during sleep (CSWDS). This condition is related to LKS.

It is important to note that conditions that mimic autism may at times coexist with autism making the diagnostic process a challenge.

Parental profiling is also very important when it comes to evaluating autism and may provide important diagnostic clues which can be useful for appropriate treatment. Patterns that I have noted in parents of children with autism include:

• Introverted shy/passive/laid back father

• Introverted mother with mild autistic symptoms, sometimes during childhood only

• Primary anxiety and or mood disorder in the mother

• Primary anxiety and or mood disorder in the father

In a family where anxiety or mood problems are prevalent on one or both sides of the family, this should be considered when designing a treatment protocol for the child. Biologically, one would search for a particular neurochemical defect that might cause these symptoms. Psychosocial concerns would also be important in that an anxious parent might impact the child's behavior inadvertently. Medical and parental profiling then should be considered since this can help the clinician focus their treatment options based on the particular needs of the individual child. Several diagnostic tools have been developed that take into account, or measure the level of stress present in the family since this will impact the child's condition.

Autism is an all encompassing disorder with a variety of symptoms seen in other neuropsychiatric conditions. There is a significant group of children with autism, for instance, that have Attention Deficit Hyperactivity Disorder (ADHD). Another important subset of children with autism and Asperger syndrome has tic disorders. A tic disorder when chronic (over a year) and when presenting with both vocal and motor symptoms is called Tourette's syndrome. Tourette's syndrome commonly presents with ADHD symptoms. Autism, Tourette's syndrome, and ADHD share many common features, have a male predominance, and are on the rise. They may actually be part of one spectrum.

A controversial set of disorders that has been described is pediatric autoimmune neuropsychiatric disorders associated with streptococcal infection, or PANDAS. This condition is mentioned here because it ties together a set of neuropsychiatric conditions including tic disorders, obsessive compulsive disorder (OCD) and ADHD that have an underlying immune component, notably an abnormal immune response following a streptococcal infection. This raises the issue of a possible immune disturbance in some neuropsychiatric conditions. Some clinicians now refer to autism as an autoimmune disorder, at least in a subset of children.

Finally, one has to consider the role of seizures. Many children with autism have seizures (see Chapter 4). The presence of seizures means that autism is associated with a specific neurologic dysfunction (brain irritability), and that there must be some significant insult to the brain to cause these seizures. We will later explore what causes the insults.

Key Points

- Autism is not one condition but a distinct group of disorders that share core clinical features.

- Autism can present from early infancy or later, but usually before the age of 3.

- Some children are severely affected and others have mild symptoms. Children with autism can have normal intelligence, mental retardation, or above normal intelligence.

- Various neuropsychiatric disorders share common features including attention deficit hyperactivity disorder, autism, obsessive compulsive disorder and Tourette's syndrome. They may all fit into one spectrum.

- There are many biological or psychological disturbances that can mimic autism. Some may coexist with autism.

3

CAUSES OF AUTISM

- What are the different causes of autism?

- How late can one develop autism?

- Do environmental factors play a role?

- Is there a consensus regarding vaccines and autism?

- Do nutritional factors play a role in the etiology of autism?

This chapter is very important because any hope of properly treating children with autism must be predicated on a proper understanding of the causes and contributing factors of autism. Autism is a multifactorial disorder. Its etiology includes genetic, metabolic-nutritional, and post-traumatic factors (the trauma being some external insult). Because the causes of autism are so diverse, it should be viewed at a *syndrome.* This means that various sets of problems that are divergent, can result in the disorder or condition we label as autism.

Any human has the potential to develop autism if the conditions are right. To develop autism you need:

1- A genetic predisposition

Instead of one gene, there are likely a set of genes that must be affected. Some children who do not qualify for a diagnosis of autism but who have a few autistic traits may have one or two affected genes. These individuals may have inherited traits such as *toe-walking, auditory defensiveness/sensory processing dysfunction, anxiety/mood dysfunction, shyness,* or *sensitivity to casein or gluten.* There may be a threshold of genetic dysfunction that must be reached for autistic symptoms to become manifest. In some cases, a specific genetic abnormality may be found.

Autism is so diverse that it may be futile though to chase after 'the autism gene'. Instead, our efforts should be directed toward looking for gene clusters and how they relate to environmental triggers in the development of autism.

2- A trigger, trauma, or insult

A trauma, trigger, or insult can occur from various sources: a viral infection, environmental pollutant, or endogenous toxins. These endogenous toxins can result from the accumulation of chemicals owing to a metabolic disorder. The trigger may not always be obvious. The 'dose' or intensity of the trigger needed will vary between individuals based on the level of inherited vulnerability. There may be one big insult or several smaller ones that have a cumulative effect leading to clinical significance. An insult may also include <u>psychogenic</u> triggers. The net effect of the insult is a disturbance in various regulatory systems of the body, most notably the immune, nervous, and gastrointestinal systems. Each system is affected to varying degrees depending on the type of insult and genetic constitution of the individual.

3- Proper timing of the insult

The insult must occur early, affecting the developing brain, starting from in-utero up until approximately 3 years of age. Leading behavioral neuroscientists such as Dr. Jocelyn Bachevalier have shown that early brain damage in specific areas can result in deleterious brain reorganization that can later lead to disorders such as autism. Depending on the level of genetic vulnerability, the intensity of the traumatizing insult, and **'other factors'**, one may have mild, moderate or severe autism, with or without mental retardation. One can have severe autistic symptoms yet be of normal intelligence or an individual can have mild autistic symptoms with co-existing mental retardation. The mental retardation may or may not be related to the autism. What are the **'other factors'** that are important in determining the phenotype of autism? The other factors that are important include:

- Co-existence of a medical disorder

- Overall early health status

- Nutritional status

- Perinatal complications

- Level of family support

- Psychosocial and stress factors

- Parental approach to health

Autism is a **developmental** disorder specifically because the triggering insult is time-dependent (i.e. it must occur before the age of three). One of the difficulties in autism is that the nature of the trigger or insult is not always apparent. The exact timing of the insult is also often unclear. There are other conditions that occur later in life that are age-dependent and may at least in part share some etiologic factors with autism. Schizophrenia and Alzheimer's disease, for instance, are two disorders, like autism, that generally start at a specific time, usually later on in life (during early and late adulthood respectively).

One factor that deserves our attention with respect to autism is nutrition. There are growing numbers of studies and reports that show a variety of nutritional and dietary abnormalities in children with autism and other neuropsychiatric conditions. Nutrient deficiencies have been documented such as zinc deficiency. Food sensitivities affect these children in various ways. Nutritional factors can have both primary and secondary roles in children with autism. For instance, an underlying nutritional-metabolic dysfunction may cause certain autistic symptoms. On the other hand, a neurological abnormality may result in feeding difficulties that can contribute to a nutritional deficiency state that can aggravate symptoms already manifest.

The diet of many children with autism is undeniably a significant problem that is often overlooked or sometimes underestimated. This diet is largely characterized by highly processed foods devoid of nutrients necessary for proper brain development, immunologic support, and overall health maintenance. There is excessive intake of refined sugar, artificial additive containing, and vitamin-antioxidant-fiber-deprived foods. THAT IS A HORRIBLE PROBLEM! Most children are also addicted to caffeinated beverages and milk. They drink very little water. This sort of diet will eventually cause a decrease in their immune defense system. In June 2002, JAMA reported: "Most people do not consume an optimal amount of all vitamins by diet alone…it appears prudent for all adults to take vitamin supplements." This statement should also include children. They are even more vulnerable than adults because of their developing brain and other organs that require proper alimentation. In addition to vitamins, various other essential nutrients should be supplemented because they are lacking (see appendix B). Our foods are becoming increasingly processed. There are growing numbers of artificial food additives that diminish the quality of our food, and ultimately our health. Let us look at just one food substance that can cause a lot of problems and typifies the idea of food toxicology (i.e. toxicological effects from the foods we eat). It is heralded by many as nutritious, wholesome, necessary and natural. Many crave it. I am referring to milk and dairy products.

There are at least 10 reasons why milk is not good for children with autism:

1. It can be highly allergenic, causing

    a. Diarrhea

    b. Eczema

    c. Recurrent attacks of nasal congestion

    d. Recurrent bronchitis

2. Many children may not be able to digest milk protein (casein)

3. Some have lactose intolerance

4. It can cause iron-deficiency anemia

5. It is associated with so-called "growing pains"

6. It can cause recurrent rashes

7. It may cause severe constipation

8. It is associated with asthma

9. In some cases it is associated with nephrosis

10. It may be contaminated with hormones and antibiotics.

It is interesting to note that cow's milk is recommended by pediatricians to be introduced in the diet of children at age one. Children with autism are perhaps more likely than most children to experience the side effects of milk due to their genetic vulnerabilities. Can it be that milk with its inherent problems can trigger a cascade of disturbances that play a significant role in autism? Is there credible evidence that milk and milk products may be harmful?

Many well-known figures including pediatricians and allergists have written about the problems with milk. One such individual is Dr. Frank Oski who wrote the book *"Don't Drink Your Milk"*. Like many, he writes that cow milk is for baby calves and can cause harm in humans. Side effects may range from mild to severe. Dr. Oski has been Professor and Chairmen of several pediatric departments including the esteemed Johns Hopkins Children's Center. He has authored hundreds of articles and written several books. He has served on the editorial board of several pediatric journals and was the founding editor of *Contemporary Pediatrics*. A physician and pediatrician of that caliber is part of the growing rank of experts that believe that dairy products can cause more harm than good.

Several medical reports have shown that a casein allergy, if present, can cause serious problems. Many children with autism have low zinc levels. Zinc is required for the peptidase enzymes that breakdown casein. It is believed and documented by studies that improperly digested casein will result in peptides called casomorphine. Casomorphine has opiate affects on the brain. This may account, in part, for the increased pain threshold, sensory processing abnormalities, aggressive behavior and "brain fog" commonly encountered in children with autism. There are a plenty of healthy alternatives to dairy (see appendix A).

Although nutritional factors may be critical as contributing factors in the etiology of autism, there are other biological and non-biological factors that should also be considered. These are discussed in the final chapter of the book. There are many conditions that are associated with autism as listed below. That is why it is always very important to have a thorough medical evaluation for a child with autism. Some of these conditions require close monitoring.

CONDITIONS THAT ARE ASSOCIATED WITH AUTISM

- Neurocutaneous disorders

  - Tuberous Sclerosis

  - Neurofibromatosis (rarely)

  - Hypomelanosis of Ito

- Congenital endocrine dysfunctions

  - Hypothyroidism

  - Juvenile diabetes

  - Pituitary deficiency

- Congenital hydrocephalus

- Neonatal infections causing encephalitis

  - Rubella

  - Cytomegalovirus

  - Herpes

- Sensory disturbances

  - Deafness

  - Partial blindness

  - Congenital anophthalmos

- Various neurometabolic disorders including:

  - Phenylketonuria (PKU)—untreated

  - Purine/pyrimidine disorders

- Various genetics disorders

  - Fragile X (most common)

Key Points

- Three conditions are required for the development of autism: a genetic predisposition, a traumatizing insult or environmental trigger, and proper timing.

- Apart from genes, there are additional aggravating factors that contribute to autism. Autism is therefore a multifactorial syndrome.

- No single gene can account for autism in most cases.

- There are genetic susceptibilities that predispose a person to the clinical manifestations of autism.

- Dietary factors play an important role in the symptomatology of autism.

- Immune and gastrointestinal factors also play a role in autism.

4

NEUROLOGICAL PERSPECTIVES ON AUTISM

- Is autism a neurological disorder?

- What part of the brain is affected in autism?

- How common are seizures in autism?

- Is autism fundamentally a sensory processing disorder?

- What neurological factors are responsible for speech and language problems in autism?

Neurological basis of autism

Is autism a neurological disorder? The answer may seem obvious today, but it is not necessarily straightforward. The most prevalent theory of autism in the past, as mentioned in the first chapter, was Bettelheims' psychogenic theory. The current neurobiological understanding of autism is as follows: During early brain development, a genetically-determined dysregulation of brain growth occurs. This dysregulation is characterized by abnormal starting and stopping of growth in neurons and supportive brain tissue. This occurs at a time that is critical for future integration of various neurocognitive functions. The dysregulation eventually leads to miswiring of the brain cells. This in turn, results in premature overgrowth of cells in some areas of the brain and reduced growth in others. This pathologic process is also believed to lead to other neurodevelopmental conditions such as dyslexia and schizophrenia. In short: early brain cell regulation problems → abnormal neurocircuitry in the developing brain → clinical manifestations of autism. Many children with autism have seizures (see below). **Seizures**

are a hallmark of cortical brain dysfunction. Therefore, we know that autism is a neurological disorder.

Neuroanatomy of autism

What parts of the brain are affected in autism? Let us subject the problem of autism to an analysis the way neurologists usually approach neurological disorders. The first question that neurologists ask is: *Where is the lesion?* This is a good question to ask because if a person presents with a sudden onset of aphasia (inability to speak) a neurologist may suspect a dominant frontal lobe stroke. On the other hand, if speech is preserved but comprehension is impaired, the neurologist might suspect a stroke in the temporal lobe.

In the case of autism, what is the brain localization for the symptoms noted? We know that children with autism have:

- Speech problems

- Comprehension or receptive language difficulties

- Involuntary movements or self-stimulatory behaviors

- Aggressive behavior

- Social interaction deficits

- Sensory processing difficulties (tactile, visual, auditory and vestibular)

- ADHD symptoms

- Seizures

Temporal lobe

Children with autism have receptive language problems as well as auditory processing disturbances. Other problems include mood disorders, aggressive behavior, irritability, and easy distractibility. All of these problems point to a temporal lobe defect since this lobe is involved in processing of auditory input. It also contains the *limbic system* which is very important in modulating emotional behavior. The mesial portion of the temporal lobe (inside section) is the most epileptogenic (seizure producing) part of the brain. As we have mentioned, seizures are common in autism. NIH studies by Mishkin and Bachevalier have in fact shown striking autistic-like behaviors following bilateral lesions of these structures in neonatal monkeys.

Frontal lobe

Many children with autism seem unable to speak, or to get the words out. Some autistic individuals who have become verbal report that prior to becoming verbal they could not figure out how to speak. Lesions or abnormalities found in the inferior part of the dominant frontal lobe result in apraxia of speech. The orbito-frontal portion of the frontal lobe can result in impulsive behavior, euphoria, emotional lability, poor judgment or insight, and distractibility. Lesions in other portions of the frontal lobe are responsible for mutism (repetition may be preserved) and outbursts of aggressive behavior.

Parietal lobe

This is often called the sensory cortex. Sensory processing difficulties are common in autism suggesting a parietal lobe dysfunction. A parietal lobe dysfunction can also result in apraxia, including a special type of apraxia called buccofacial apraxia where there is impaired control of facial and mouth movements.

Temporo-parietal cortex

The junction between the temporal and parietal lobes is where auditory information (a temporal lobe function) and sensory functions (from the parietal lobe) come together. As such, this is a part of the brain that is responsible for processing auditory sensory information at a higher level. This area allows an individual to make sense of an experience that has been captured through the sense of hearing. In the case of autism, a young child may hear his name called, but he may not be able to attach the right meaning to that sound and thus may not respond appropriately when his name is called.

It is very revealing that conditions such as Landau-Kleffner syndrome, which can mimic autism in symptomatology, affect this particular portion of the brain (see further discussion in the seizure section below).

Subcortical structures

Subcortical brain structures are ones that occur in the lower part of the brain. Examples include the basal ganglia, hypothalamus, other diencephelic structures, and the brainstem. These structures participate in certain aspects of speech, arousal mechanisms, emotional behavior, affect, repetitive behaviors, and regulation of sleep, temperature and the autonomic system.

Other parts of the brain have also been implicated in autism such as the occipital lobe, which is the visual cortex and the cerebellum which is important for coordination and may be involved in certain aspects of language.

So again the question is: where is the lesion? Based on the above discussion, it would seem that the lesion can be almost anywhere. In vivo radiographic studies show that several areas of the brain can be affected: the limbic system, the cerebellum, and several other areas. In one important study done in Japan in 2000 (reported in Brain vol. 123, No 9, 1938—1844) Ohnishi et al. used SPECT scans to demonstrate decreased blood flow to the bilateral insula, superior temporal gyri, left inferior frontal gyrus and left middle frontal gyrus. Other studies have shown involvement in other areas, and one earlier French study also using SPECT studies showed no cortical involvement at all. It appears, based on the above discussion that there are a variety of areas that can be affected in autism. Consider the problem of attention span, which is seen in most children with autism. Disturbances in attention can be caused by problems in the frontal cortex (prefrontal area), temporoparietal cortex, limbic system and some subcortical areas. This means that attention problems likely involve different parts of the brain.

What does all of this mean? It seems obvious that various parts of the brain can be implicated clinically as well as radiographically. Instead of one localized lesion, we must instead consider the existence of a diffuse lesion. This pattern usually fits a toxic-metabolic profile. If a child has a metabolic or toxic disturbance, one would expect different areas of the brain to be affected although particular areas may be more vulnerable than others.

When a neurologist is confronted with a problem that cannot be localized to one area but that still appears neurological, that neurologist considers the possibility of an autoimmune disorder, such as multiple sclerosis (MS). Autism, in many cases, may well be a form of an autoimmune disorder, like MS. I believe then that instead of permanent focal brain damage, in many cases we are dealing with a dysfunction affecting several parts of the brain that with early, proper, and aggressive treatment may be reversed.

Pathophysiology of autism

Neuropathological studies have shown that a mechanism of brain injury in children with autism is that of neuroinflammation (i.e. inflammation of brain tissues). One recent study reported in a November 15, 2004 article of the *Annals of Neurology* showed the presence of neuroglial activation and neuroinflammation in the brains of individuals with autism. The investigators had studied the brain tissue of 11 autistic individuals aged 4—44 that died due to accidents or injuries. This study was done at Johns Hopkins Medical Center in Baltimore. The main question is where does the inflammation come from and what are the implications? Possible options would include a toxic source, a neurometabolic defect, an autoimmune disturbance, or a cascade of events that includes all of the above.

One theory is that of toxic insult from substances such as mercury. Mercury is known to be toxic to the brain, especially the developing brain. Many researchers, including toxicologists believe that there is a connection between mercury neurotoxicity and the development of autism and other neurodevelopmental disorders. Mercury can come from a variety of sources such as Thimerosal (which is a mercury-containing preservative that has been used in some vaccines), mercury-based dental amalgams, contaminated fish, and environmental sources. Can increased mercury exposure account for the epidemic explosion of autism and other neuropsychiatric disorders? That difficult question and other controversial issues are addressed in Chapter 26.

As far as the clinical manifestations of autism and other conditions such as ADHD and Tourette's syndrome, some researchers believe that there may be blood flow and oxygen—dependent abnormalities resulting in abnormal brain function. This has led some clinicians to the use pharmacological drugs (vasodilators) and non-pharmacological approaches (hyperbaric oxygen treatment) that enhance blood flow and oxygenation to the brain (see further discussion in Chapter 20).

Seizures in Autism and other Neurological Disorders

We know that autism is a neurological disorder because of the high incidence of seizures in children with autism. **Unprovoked recurrent seizures are always a hallmark of cortical brain dysfunction**. In the general population the incidence of epilepsy is approximately 0.5%. The incidence of seizures in autism was traditionally found to be approximately 30%. More recent studies that take into consideration the most advanced form of electroencephalogram called MEG (magnetoencephalography), suggests that the incidence is much higher. If you combine children with EEG abnormalities with those that also have clinical epileptic manifestations, the incidence of seizures increases from 30% to over 80%.

There are two peak occurrences for the onset of seizures in autistic children. The first peak is during the toddler years and the second during adolescence. I speculate that toddlers may start having seizures because of developmental changes in the brain combined with accumulating toxic or nutritional factors which aggravate the brain. In adolescence, the manifestation of seizures may in part be related to developmental changes in the brain coupled with hormonal factors.

Definition of seizures and difference between seizures and epilepsy

Seizures are intermittent, temporary disturbances that can affect motor, sensory, behavioral, autonomic or mental functions. These disturbances are caused by an underlying electrical discharge (electrical storm) in the brain. Although given the right set of circumstances (e.g. extreme sleep depravation) anyone can have <u>one</u> seizure, recurrent seizures however signal a dysfunction of the cerebral cortex (outer portion of the brain tissue). When someone has more than one <u>unprovoked</u> seizure, that individual has epilepsy. Epilepsy then is a condition where, due to cortical brain dysfunction someone is prone to having recurrent seizures. Although I have used the term 'unprovoked', in reference to epilepsy, there is always some type of trigger (see appendix G). The term 'unprovoked' is used to exclude non-neurologic factors such as electrolyte disturbances. Individuals for instance, who develop hypoglycemia (low blood sugar) and subsequently develop a seizure, do not have epilepsy if the recurrent seizures are due to hypoglycemic episodes.

Seizures can be **PARTIAL** if they are caused by a <u>focal</u> electrical storm or **GENERALIZED** if the <u>entire</u> brain is affected <u>simultaneously</u>. Partial seizures can further be subdivided into simple partial meaning that the seizures <u>do not affect awareness or responsiveness</u>. An example of simple partial seizures would include a child who has jerking of the face or arm, but is still aware of his surroundings and responsive during the episode. Simple partial seizures may sometimes be confused with motor tics or psychogenic (non-epileptic) seizures. Complex partial seizures are ones where consciousness is affected to a certain degree. Some of these seizures may present with a brief vacant stare. Other complex partial seizures can occur with rapid eye fluttering for a brief period of time with some alteration in consciousness. Yet other seizures can present with a period of confusion or dazed behavior without any motor manifestations. Some children with unrecognized complex partial seizures have been described as frequently ignoring others or being stubborn. These children while they are staring may be experiencing brief lapses in consciousness related to seizures that prevents them from responding. There are also unsuspecting types of seizures such laughing (gelastic) seizures, crying seizures, and running in circle or *cursive* seizures (see appendix F).

The other major type of seizures fall under the category of generalized seizures. Most people when they think of seizures visualize individuals having full body jerking and stiffening with foaming at the mouth, biting of the tongue and upward rolling of the eyes. This is what some refer to as *grand mal* seizures (as opposed to more subtle *petit mal seizures*). Neurologists prefer the more specific term *generalized tonic-clonic seizures*. The term *petit mal* is not a good term because it is non-specific. Petit mal seizures may refer to complex partial seizures (which are focal in nature) or absence seizures (which are brief and subtle but generalized).

Seizures can be preceded by an *aura* which is a sort of warning sign that indicates that a person is about to have a seizure. This can be an abnormal feeling in the gut or some strange behavior. Auras are usually very stereotypical and precede seizures by only a few minutes. Following a seizure, the individual (depending on the type of seizure and its duration) may be very sleepy, confused or disoriented. We refer to these symptoms as *postictal* manifestations.

Diagnostic relevance of seizures in autistic disorders

We have spent a lot of time discussing seizures because they are a very important consideration in autism and neuropsychiatric disorders. Seizures must always be suspected and treated when found. Untreated seizures can affect cognition and lead to a variety of secondary problems. As far as autism is concerned, the presence of seizures brings out a lot of important considerations. Let us suppose that autism was first diagnosed in the context of neurology instead of psychiatry, how would that affect the current theories and treatment options for autism?

To answer that question, let us look at the condition known as Landau-Kleffner syndrome (LKS). LKS was first reported in a neurology journal by Dr. William Landau and Dr. Frank Kleffner in 1957. They described a condition where an association was made between 'acquired aphasia' and 'convulsive disorder in children'. Landau-Kleffner syndrome (LKS) is a condition that highly resembles autism but usually has a later onset (usually age 3–7 years in typical cases). EEG abnormalities, pure word agnosia and other clinical findings point to an abnormality in the temporo-parietal cortex, although EEG abnormalities may be multifocal. This *autistic-like* condition is usually classified as a neurological disorder because of the presence of seizures and the uniform presence of EEG abnormalities. Like most autistic disorders, there is a male predominance. Many neurologists classify this disorder as a form of acquired epileptic aphasia (AEA), and place it under the general rubric of *electrical status epilepticus of sleep* (ESES). Some children may have EEG abnormalities only when they enter deep sleep and then the EEG may be almost continuously abnormal (more than 85% of the sleep period). Incidentally, there is a subgroup of children with autism that have what neurologists call LKS-variant. LKS may actually be on the same continuum as autism and, as far as I am concerned, should be classified in the category of autistic spectrum disorders. A subset of children with autism may share the same underlying dysfunction as those with LKS, usually a neuro-autoimmune disturbance. These children, instead of responding to anticonvulsant medication, usually do better with immune modulating agents (such as ACTH, steroids or IVIG). In refractory cases, more invasive interventions have been considered for LKS such as the neurosurgical technique of multiple subpial resections.

There are important lessons to learn from Landau-Kleffner syndrome. It may be a perfect model or prototype of an acquired, neuro-autoimmune, seizure-related autistic disorder. What this means, in a practical sense, is that any child with regressive symptoms who is nonverbal, whether or not there are obvious signs of seizures, should have an EEG to determine whether underlying seizures may be present. Immune modulating treatment should be considered.

An EEG should be an important part of the evaluation of individuals with autistic disorders. The EEG though has certain limitations since it is a snapshot picture in time of brain wave activity. Someone who is having seizures but who is having them very intermittently may not always have a signature abnormality seen on EEG. This is especially the case with a routine EEG where no drowsiness or sleep is obtained. For this reason it is always important to acquire a sleep-deprived EEG, especially when seizures are strongly suspected and a previous awake-only EEG has been reported as normal. In some cases one may need a more prolonged study such as a 24 hour ambulatory or overnight EEG. Some abnormalities are only seen during deep sleep. The possibility of seizures should always be considered since seizures, when present, can affect behavior, cognitive development and communication skills. In some cases, seizures may directly relate to lack of speech (epileptic aphasia). Seizure medicines are prescribed based on the type of seizure present. As in the case of LKS, some children with autism who have seizures may only respond to immune therapies.

AUTISM AS A SENSORY PROCESSING DISORDER

Auditory defensiveness

This is one of the most pervasive and often overlooked problems in ASD. Many children with ASD have hyperacute or painful hearing. They can often perceive sounds that normal people cannot. These children, for instance, may hear an approaching airplane long before other people. Unfortunately, various sounds can be very annoying to them and can affect their behavior. In my experience, I have noted that many of these children have coexisting central auditory processing disorders. It appears that their auditory acuity is over developed, perhaps at the expense of normal auditory processing and comprehension. There are various auditory based therapies that are aimed at desensitizing their hearing (see Chapter 22). Hopefully, helping with auditory processing and related auditory dysfunction can improve behavior, socialization and other areas of deficit.

Tactile defensiveness

Many children with ASD feel uncomfortable when they are touched in certain areas of their bodies. Some children, for this reason do not like to be held and may clearly withdraw from hugs and other acts of affection. One high functioning adolescent boy with ASD explained to me that receiving a hug felt like a ton of bricks falling on him, even when from his mother. Just as in the case of auditory perceptions, where hearing may be painful, certain tactile stimulation can be very uncomfortable and may in part explain some of the behaviors noted. Difficulty with eating can also relate to oral defensiveness from the inability to tolerate certain textures of food.

Visual processing defects

Vision can be distorted in a variety of neurological and psychiatric conditions including: migraine headaches, Alice-in-wonderland syndrome (where objects have distorted sizes), seizures (where the visual cortex is affected), strokes (where the parieto-occipital cortex is involved), intoxicated states (endogenous or exogenous), and psychosis. The same may apply in some cases of autism. Various objects may appear distorted. In other cases there is some form of light sensitivity. One may have dyslexia or visual agnosia (seeing something without attaching the right meaning, such as a person's face that is viewed as an inanimate object). At least in some cases, these visual perceptual abnormalities may account for the strange manner in which some children with autism look from the corner of their eyes repeatedly. Some children with ASD are apparently able to perceive certain visual phenomena such as a 60 hertz cycle from a light bulb, and fluorescent lighting can be very annoying to them unbeknownst to others. Behavioral optometrists may be able to help with some of these disorders even when a formal eye exam is normal.

Attention deficit hyperactive disorder (ADHD)

Attention deficit hyperactivity disorder can be viewed as a form of sensory processing abnormality. Individuals with an attention deficit may not be able to filter out non useful, trivial, or irrelevant stimuli. There is concomitant distractibility. Attention may be so short that it directly affects other areas of behavior such as socialization. For example, the attention given to another person's face or eyes may be so short as to give the appearance of having poor eye contact or eye avoidance. Learning may also be affected. Many children with ASD may come to medical attention, initially, because they are hyperactive and inattentive. Unfortunately, there are many children who are diagnosed late because they come to medical attention specifically for ADHD. While some children have symptoms that respond to stimulants, it is important to be extremely cautious with the use of stimulants in this group. Some children with ASD can have the opposite effect when stimulants are given. Some who also have an underlying tendency or predisposition for tics may have a drastic exacerbation of these symptoms if placed on stimulants. As with other conditions, it is best to identify the patient's nutritional and metabolic status and to make sure that he/she is properly supplemented and is eating a wholesome diet. This should be a priority. In many instances one will find a great improvement with the ADHD symptoms just as with other autistic problems when diet and nutrition are properly adjusted.

Central auditory processing disorder (CAPD)

A distortion in sounds from spoken language can have grave consequences. Imagine that you have perfect hearing, but that you cannot make proper sense of what you have heard. In some cases, one may take a very long time to comprehend what is said instead of comprehending immediately. The processing of auditory information may be very slow. In other cases, one may hear something slightly different from what was actually said, resulting in confusion. We have found that children with auditory processing difficulties often have ADHD and hyperacusis (or painful hearing). In the case of hyperacusis, this can be so unbearable that the young child learns to tune out certain sounds simply as a coping mechanism. Hence, the child appears deaf when not responding to certain sounds, although formal testing reveals normal hearing. CAPD should not be confused with mental retardation. Many individuals with or without autism may have some degree of CAPD with normal or above normal intelligence. As always, identifying and treating the underlying problem is important and can greatly improve the quality of life for the child.

Sensory processing abnormalities should always be considered in the child with autism and addressed if found. When it is properly identified and dealt with, the quality of life may greatly be enhanced.

Lock-in syndrome

Given all of the above problems present, autism can be viewed as a sort of "Locked-in syndrome". Locked-in syndrome is a neurological condition caused by a devastating stroke or trauma affecting particular parts of the brain. A victim is left without the ability to move, communicate, or respond even though the mind is intact. Such individuals only retain the ability to control closure of the eye. This is their only mode of communication. Similarly, with severe autism a child may be "locked-in". Although the mind may be intact in autism, there are various barriers that *lock these children in*. These barriers are disturbances in sensory, linguistic, behavioral and social functioning. Although speech and language difficulties are significant barriers in autism, sensory processing abnormalities can be just as important. Sensory disturbances, in particular hearing distortions or perceptual abnormalities can contribute to many of the limitations seen in autism. Some odd behaviors may actually represent adaptive ways of altering sensory function, whether it is auditory, visual or tactile, to cope with and try to better understand the external environment. Imagine what life would be like if everything other people said sounded like a foreign language. You too would appear socially aloof with altered responsiveness. If you heard explosive sounds, you might have a tendency to cover your ears. The senses are in fact the "avenue to the soul". Visual, auditory, tactile, gustatory and olfactory distortions can affect one's interaction with, and perception of the outside world.

Other neurological problems in ASD and neuropsychiatric disorders

Headaches

Headaches are likely to occur in a large number of children with ASD including those that are too young to complain or those that are nonverbal and cannot express this symptom in a meaningful way. A lot of children with ASD have genetic, nutritional, toxic, metabolic, and personality traits that make them prone to migraine headaches. Autistic children that have severe and prolonged crying fits should be evaluated for the possibility of headaches.

Starting from a very young age children who otherwise appear normal can suffer from migraine headaches. *Migraine equivalents* are symptoms encountered in children (with or without autism) that can be an early indication for the development of full-blown migraines headaches later in their life. These migraine equivalents are symptoms that are thought to be related to migraines without the actual presence of a headache. These symptoms include:

- Recurrent vomiting episodes (sometimes called cyclic vomiting)

- Bouts of spontaneous ambulatory instability or ataxia (sometimes associated with a condition called benign paroxysmal vertigo)

- Confusional states that can resemble complex seizures and may last several hours

- Various autonomic disturbances such as temporary pupillary dilation or pallor of the skin

- Visual disturbances such as temporary blindness, double vision or distorted perception of objects (e.g. Alice-in-wonderland syndrome where objects may appear unusually large or small)

Because of the possibility of migraines, it is very important to encourage proper nutrition, hydration with **water,** and avoidance of migraine food triggers (see Appendix A). Non-nutritional triggers of migraine should also be avoided (see Appendix G).

Tourette's syndrome and Tic disorders

Tics are involuntary stereotypic movements or behaviors that tend to wax and wane. Tics can be of the motor type if there are involuntary muscle movements. Motor tics can be simple or complex. Complex motor tics include semi-purposeful movements such as squatting, jumping or other movements that are complex. Examples of simple motor tics include:

- Frequent eye blinking

- Shoulder shrugging

- Facial grimacing

Tics can also be vocal or phonic if a particular sound is produced.

Examples of simple phonic tics include:

- Grunting

- Sniffing

- Throat clearing

As you can imagine, some children who are experiencing phonic tics can sometimes end up getting an evaluation for an allergy condition. The allergy medicine prescribed of course would not be useful. Complex phonic tics are those that involve utterances and phrases. These may sometimes be offensive or inappropriate. When there are offensive utterances such as swearing or use of bad language this is called *coprolalia*. The urge to express distasteful things can also occur in other forms apart from language. In the case of written language, writing foul things is referred to as *coprographia*. *Copropraxia* refers to affectively inappropriate use of obscene gestures. Some speculate that Mozart the musician had coprographia. When a child has a variety of both motor and phonic tics and that these have been present (intermittently) for more than a year, the child can be diagnosed with **Tourette's syndrome.**

It is interesting to note that a significant subset of individuals with autism, especially those who are high functioning, have tics. In some cases, the tics may be so conspicuous that the individuals receive a label of Tourette's syndrome, when in reality they have autism (or Asperger syndrome) with the coexistence of tics. It is important to realize that there is a definite connection between ASD and Tourette's syndrome. Both conditions are predominant in males. Both conditions often present with ADHD. Both conditions have associated anxiety and obsessive-compulsive symptoms. Both conditions may include echolalia, palilalia, and echopraxia. Many children with Tourette's syndrome have a variety of sensory processing disturbances including problems with delayed cognitive processing. Many children have rage attacks and other behavioral problems. Tourette's syndrome should be included in the ASD category because it shares many symptoms with autism, and the underlying pathology may be similar.

Lack of coordination

Some children with ASD are clumsy, although they may have great intellectual and cognitive abilities. There are a variety of reasons why coordination can be impaired: low muscle tone, loose or hypermobile joints, metabolic/nutritional derangements, or subtle structural brain defects. Many children have difficulties with fine motor skills even if their gross motor skills appear adequate. A good example is handwriting, which can be a problem for many children with ASD. If a child also has coexisting obsessive-compulsive tendencies, which is common, writing can be very difficult. Some children with obsessive-compulsive tendencies are also perfectionists, and tend to rewrite over what they have already written repeatedly. Given that their handwriting is poor or that they may hate writing, this can make any written homework assignments laborious. I believe that with proper overall treatment of the autistic symptoms, coordination will improve.

Sleep disturbance

Many children with ASD do not sleep well. There are a variety of factors that may explain why sleep is impaired. One is nocturnal reflux, headaches, stomachaches, or hormonal/endocrine problems such as low production of melatonin. All of these conditions can interfere with sleep. In some cases anxiety, stress, or certain sounds (inaudible to others) can also contribution to sleep disturbances (see appendix E).

Problems with speech/language/communication

Children with autism by definition have problems with communication. This includes both receptive language (comprehension) and expressive language (speech). Keep in mind that there is a broad range in the severity of abnormalities seen in autism. This means that some children on the higher end of the spectrum may have relatively mild communication impairment while others, on the lower end, may be severely affected with complete mutism and apparent lack of any comprehension. Even children with high functioning autism who appear to speak very well with excellent elocution may still have subtle language difficulties and deficits. These may include problems with conversational language. They may have difficulties responding to questions in an elaborate way. Language may be one-sided and overly focused on the individual's particular set of interests, which may be narrow but profound. There can be deficits in voice inflection and pitch.

Many parents note that language and speech deficits may fluctuate. Even in relatively non-verbal individuals, there may be periods where spontaneous words or phrases emerge, though inconsistently. There may be unpredictable periods of lucidity where comprehension seems better. Along with this variation of speech and language, many autistic children are noted to have unusually strong wills, are stubborn, and like to have things done their way on their terms. In some emotional states, speech, behavior and cognitive function seem to fluctuate at times to amazing levels. This raises two questions: the role of emotional states and cognitive level of functioning in autism, and the difference between what children with autism will not and cannot do. In this section, we will only address the "can't" of autism with respective to language.

Many children with autism want to speak but cannot

Many children with autism have significant speech impediments that do not allow them to express themselves verbally, although they may otherwise have normal cognitive abilities. There are various mechanisms and biological structures that have to function properly to allow speech to occur. One example would include the tongue. Someone may have the ability to speak but if the cranial nerve or neuronal pathways that control tongue movement are significantly impaired, then speech may not occur. There are cases where children with autism can "speak in their mind" but are unable to get the words out. Other individuals with autism that seem to be able to speak do so in a very low tone (hypophonic), or their articulation may be so poor that what comes out is almost unintelligible (especially to non family members).

Specifically, what are the different speech impediments that interfere with proper communication in children with ASD? In my experience, one often overlooked culprit is the presence of underlying seizures. If a child is having frequent seizures, whether they are obvious, subtle, or even subclinical (i.e. you are unable to see anything externally) that child's seizures may interfere with their ability to speak. Other neurological and cognitive functions may be affected also. Therefore, it is always very important to rule out the presence of seizures in these children. This may entail doing an electroencephalogram (EEG), although in many cases that may not be enough. As mentioned above, one may have to do a prolonged sleep-deprived EEG or even a 24-hour video EEG to determine if a child is having seizures.

What are some of the other possibilities that cause speech deficits in a child with autism? Hearing problems is always a consideration. There may be partial hearing loss or there may be a major problem interpreting what is heard (central auditory processing difficulty). In some cases, inattention may be so severe that progress in the acquisition of language is significantly impaired. An autistic child who is receiving appropriate therapies and where everything is improving significantly (including receptive language skills) but where no progress at all is made with speech, one should always consider, or rule out the presence of a structural central nervous system abnormality. Because of the possibility of seizures or an underlying structural abnormality, it is always important to consider evaluation by a child neurologist. Although a variety of specialists are able to diagnose autism, child neurologists are specially trained to assess and, if necessary, treat *neurological problems* associated with autism such as seizures.

Key Features

- Autism is a neurological disorder. The presence of seizures, language defects and other cortical abnormalities support this conclusion.

- Various parts of the brain are affected in autism. Most commonly the temporal and frontal lobes.

- There are a variety of associated neurological problems that can contribute to the overall symptomatology of autism.

- Sensory processing abnormalities play a vital role in the cognitive and behavioral manifestations of autism.

- Tourette's syndrome and ADHD should be included in the spectrum of autistic disorders.

5

PSYCHIATRIC ASPECTS OF AUTISM

- Can autism be considered a psychiatric disorder? Has it been?

- What are the psychiatric disturbances in autism?

- Are psychiatric problems directly related to the core defects in autism?

- How should psychiatric problems in autism be addressed?

- How do psychiatric problems in autism relate to other psychiatric disorders?

From the very beginning, autistic terms included psychiatric terms such as *symbiotic psychosis* and *childhood schizophrenia*. Leo Kanner, the father of autism, was himself a child psychiatrist. Currently, autism is listed in the Diagnostic and Statistical Manuel of Mental Disorders, Fourth Edition (the DSM-IV). The term used is 'Autistic Disorder' under the rubric of Pervasive Developmental Disorders and a specific psychiatric diagnostic code, recognized by insurance companies, has been assigned. By virtue of its inclusion in the DSM-IV, autism is officially a mental or psychiatric condition. I personally believe that psychiatric problems exist in autism, as I will describe below. It should not be classified as a psychiatric condition however, any more than Tourette's syndrome. Tourette's syndrome in the past was thought to be a psychiatric condition because of the partial ability to suppress tics and the bizarre nature of some of the tics. Later, Tourette's syndrome was reclassified as a neurological disorder.

Although I believe that calling autism a psychiatric disorder is misleading, there are undeniably psychiatric symptoms and factors present in children with ASD. Let us look specifically at the problem of self-stimulatory behaviors. Self-stimulation is a specific problem commonly encountered in children with ASD. Sometimes these repetitive behaviors can be so frequent and persistent that they become very annoying. Self-stimulatory behavior can include such things as rocking, flapping, twirling, looking at things from the corner of the eyes, eying things perhaps as an architect would and toe-walking, to name a few. Some self-stimulatory behaviors and movements can be bizarre. Most children with ASD have some form of repetitive behavior which, according to the context and manifestation may pertain either to what we call self-stimulatory behavior, tic disorder, or compulsion (part of obsessive compulsive behavior). These may fit in the broad category of an anxiety disorder. Certainly, when children with autism are stressed these behaviors may be exacerbated. These children can have very unusual fascinations and habits such as pica (eating objects like dirt, flowers, leaves or paper).

Self-stimulatory behaviors may be due to an:

> Anxiety disorder
> Self-soothing mechanism/coping mechanism
> Seizure (non-epileptic)
> Mode or form of communication
> Movement disorder/hyperkinesias
> Response to internal stimuli

All of the above are distinct etiological possibilities to explain self-stimulatory behaviors, and there may also be a combination of the above factors. These possibilities may coexist, and are not mutually exclusive. Motor tics, for example, have a lot in common with autistic self—stimulatory behaviors. Both may provide a comforting purpose. Both can occur intermittently. Both can occur in times of stress or boredom. Both can be exacerbated by illness, and both can drive the parents to distraction.

Most neurologists would not consider self-stimulatory behaviors as a manifestation of epileptic seizures because motor seizures that originate in the cerebral cortex are usually distinct from those seen with these behaviors. Unlike self-stimulatory behaviors, seizures are completely outside of a person's control. One way to view these behaviors, however, is to consider that self-stimulation is a form of a **non-epileptic** seizure. Instead of a structural or fixed metabolic derangement causing an irritable cortex, these children may have sub-cortical dysfunctions causing their abnormalities. These subcortical areas may be susceptible to toxins, neurochemicals, infections, and toxic overload from detoxification problems or hormonal imbalances. This produces an abnormal motor response secondary to internal stress factors.

The best way to understand self-stimulation is to view it in terms of a dysfunction of neurological, emotional, and psychological origins. This dysfunction affects movement centers in certain portions of the brain resulting in these abnormal repetitive behaviors. Parents and other caregivers must understand that, although these behaviors may occasionally be suppressed, they are primarily involuntary movements. It is also important to understand that added stress created by family members or other people, can exacerbate the self-stimulatory behaviors, just like with tics. If a child starts having self-stimulatory behaviors, the first important step is to identify what possible triggers may be causing the symptoms. Again, these triggers can be toxic, metabolic, nutritional, infectious, or emotional. This may happen if the child eats something to which the child is overly sensitive. The fact that a food substance could cause abnormal behaviors should not be too surprising since certain drugs, such as stimulant medication may also do the same in a vulnerable individual. The stressors that affect a child with autism are often not perceived by others as being relevant. There are also other possible explanations. One individual with autism wrote: "I sometimes need to flap my hands or sway my body, to find where I left it. I need to control as many things as I can to make my world as safe as possible".

AUTISM AS A MOOD DISORDER

Mood disorders, such as depression, may be severe in autism. We have previously mentioned a condition known as pseudoautism where, due to significant depression, a child may manifest symptoms of autism. If properly treated, the depression resolves, and the child no longer appears autistic. With true autism, however, many children may develop primary or secondary mood changes. In many cases, one may find a family history of mood disorder that has been inherited. There are many reasons why an autistic child may eventually develop a secondary or reactive depression with autism. Mood changes are important in that they can significantly affect behavior and cognitive performance. Mood problems should be considered and treated as fully as possible.

Key Points

- Psychiatric disturbances play a prominent role in children with autism.

- Psychiatric disturbances are commonly based on underlying biological factors.

- Although psychiatric disturbances are present, autism should not be viewed primarily as a psychiatric disorder.

- Mood disturbances are common and may affect cognitive, social, and behavioral functioning.

- Stress plays a vital role in autism and may in part explain the presentation and exacerbation of self-stimulatory behaviors.

6

THE AUTISTIC MIND

- What goes on in the mind of autistic individuals?

- What abilities do we have that autistic individuals lack?

- Can elucidation of the autistic mind solve the mind-body question?

- What is mind-blindness?

- Why do autistic individual think the way they do? Can they have unusual gifts and talents?

What goes on in the mind of autistic individuals? The following are comments made by autistic individuals who have gained the ability to speak or who can write even if they cannot communicate verbally:

- "I could talk in my mind but could not figure out how to get the words out."

- "As a child, the environment appeared chaotic and unpredictable."

- "Words are so slippery at times and the same words can mean so many different things."

- "I am a child you cannot see in the body of an adult you don't understand."

- "I get totally lost in fascination with things you never see, and often, I completely miss your smiles and your frowns."

An interesting concept that has been developed is that of "mind-blindness", and the "theory of the mind" in autism. It attempts to dissect the mental aberrations that are associated with the social defects seen in autism. Simon Baron-Cohen, Professor in Developmental Psychopathology and Director of the Autism Research Center at the University of Cambridge, discusses these concepts in his book: <u>Mind-blindness, An Essay on Autism and Theory of Mind</u>. He specifically argues that normal human beings have evolved the ability to 'mind-read' which allows us to interpret, predict and participate in social behavior and communication. Children with autism lack that ability. They are not able to interpret thoughts, emotions, and gazes, leading to a state of "mind-blindness".

If one is unable to appreciate the social nuances in linguistic and facial expression then that makes social interactions difficult. The autistic mind, although different from our own, is quite fascinating and very consistent with the behavior that they manifest. The autistic person focuses on routine, structure, symmetry, and order and has a tendency to miss the social nuances that are a part of normal human experiences.

AUTISM AS A PSYCHOGENIC DISORDER

Children with autism experience a variety of physical and psychological stresses. An interesting supposition is that some children with autism may experience symptoms that are related to a psychological trauma that occurred when they were young. Some children with autism can be described as having a form of PTSD (Post traumatic stress disorder). In the context of autism, PTSD can also stand for 'post *toxic* stress disorder'. Many children with autism can become intoxicated by various agents, environmental or dietary. This results in a chronic stressor with resultant emotional, mood, and anxiety disorders.

Some children with a particular emotional genetic predisposition may be prone to experiencing ongoing disturbances from an emotional trauma. This trauma may seem trivial to the parents or other individuals, but not to the affected child. Psychological trauma can be just as devastating as a physical trauma. Both can cause seizures, non-epileptic or epileptic. Both can affect behavior, speech, language, movement, self-stimulatory abnormalities, and social interaction. Therefore, both physical and psychological trauma require proper identification and treatment. Children with autism are usually extremely strong-willed. This may in part serve as a defense mechanism for them to help cope with the various stresses they experience.

Some children with autism may truly have psychogenic mutism where psychological disturbances prevent them from being able to speak. Others may have elective mutism where they speak only to certain individuals and under certain conditions. Of course there are many children with ASD that truly do not know how to speak as discussed in the chapter on neurological perspectives.

WON'T AND CAN'T OF AUTISM WITH RESPECT TO LANGUAGE

How much do children with autism understand? Is it possible that they understand more than we think they do? In the cases where there is absolutely no evidence of an underlying structural or biological abnormality that can account for the child's inability to speak, one has to consider the seemingly strange possibility that some children with autistic symptoms *can actually speak*, but for some reason **won't** do so.

Some children with autism do not want to speak but actually can.

Some children with autism may actually have coexisting elective mutism, or may be extremely shy. Elective mutism is a condition where an individual who has the ability to speak will do so only in certain circumstances or environments. In my practice, I have been made aware of several instances where a 'nonverbal' child who is upset or very excited about something that he wants, will actually speak in complete sentences, to everyone's surprise.

Now what would cause a child who has the ability to speak to remain mute? I believe that most of the children in this category are ones that are exceedingly strong-willed or, as some parents put it, extremely stubborn. These children may be very oppositional, defiant, and have anger problems. Some of these children may have behavioral or psychogenic impairments that cause their speech to be *suppressed*. I suggest that a subset of children with ASD have psychogenic mutism. The underlying processes that account for the behavioral difficulties and the extreme strong-will in their personality, may also account for the psychogenic mutism. There are still many things that we do not understand about the human body and especially the mind of young children. It is my belief that even young children can have behavioral and psychological/psychiatric disturbances that can affect aspects of their cognitive and behavioral function. Parents have described what appears to be clinical depression in their children. It may be difficult to visualize a depressed individual who is only 3 years old, but this is possible. The depression may result from endogenous abnormalities. There may be some intrinsic biological defect that is independent of environmental factors causing the depression. Mood disorders, including depression, may be much more prevalent in children with ASD than previously thought.

Lack of speech can also be a means of gaining control of one's surroundings. A child can get a lot of attention by not speaking, though this may be partly subconscious. A child might be able to fulfill various psychosocial needs by suppressing speech that might not be possible if speech were expressed. The underlying factors that would cause such problems in a young child would include a combination of genetic factors, endogenous biological abnormalities, environmental conditions, and the child's particular personality traits. The treatment approach for these children would be different from that applied to children who try very hard to speak but have impairments that are more organic or structural in nature.

A unique way to view the language problem in some children with ASD is to consider the presence of a severe biologically-based, psychiatric disturbance that causes a child to be extremely oppositional, defiant, strong-willed, obsessive-compulsive, moody and quick to anger. In this context, speech, or lack thereof, can be used as a strong agent of manipulation. There are many children with ASD, however, that are severely affected and truly cannot speak and may not show an outward desire to do so because of the underlying severity of their condition. These children may have varying degrees of cognitive dysfunction and delays.

Many children who are neglected or abused may also display autistic features. Fortunately, they may have chronic problems that are completely reversible in the proper environment. This tells us that mind and brain interactions are dynamic and marvelously interconnected. A neglected child can be forced to turn inward as a coping mechanism, and may eventually develop autistic traits. It is known that many institutionalized children demonstrate autistic behaviors. The formative years are very important for future psychological adjustment in life. Young children, like adults, may be susceptible to psychogenic disturbances that can in part, result in autistic symptomatology.

SOCIAL DEFICTS

One of the most consistent and profoundly abnormal problems in autism is that of social interaction. Social interaction deficits are often severe, even in autistic individuals with above normal intelligence. There are two main presentations for social interaction deficits that we encounter in individuals with autism. In the first category, children are very aloof and are content to be by themselves. This is what led to Leo Kanner's use of the term *autistic aloneness*. Autistic people do not seem interested in other individuals. They seem quite able to entertain themselves. These individuals, as young children, show little affection even toward close family members. They may spend hours in their own world. Along with the social aloofness, these children have endless repetitive movements. In his original paper, Leo Kanner stated: "we must then assume that these children have come into this world with innate inability to form the usual, biologically provided affective contact with people just as others come into this world with physical or intellectual handicaps".

Why do the children in the first category prefer to be by themselves? There are many factors that come into play that do not allow these children to interact meaningfully with their surroundings. For instance, if this is a child with very severe auditory processing difficulties, including the constant experiencing of painful auditory stimuli, that child will subconsciously learn to shut himself off from the external environment as a coping mechanism. That child will then be forced to turn inward and focus on his internal stimuli. These stimuli may be thoughts, images, recorded phrases from TV recalled with stunning accuracy or other internal signals. As you can imagine, it would be very difficult for a child who is unable to appropriately make sense of the external environment, to socially interact as a normal person. As you might also suspect, the more profound the sensory processing defect, the more significant will be the lack of reciprocal social interaction.

In the second category of social interaction deficit, a subset of children with autism actually seem desirous of interacting with others but obviously still lack the appropriate social skills to do so properly. These children usually are of higher cognitive functioning and will often attempt to be around other individuals. Because they lack very important social cues that make proper reciprocal social interaction possible, their attempts may fail leaving them frustrated, discouraged, and sometimes depressed. These individuals may completely lack tact and inadvertently make comments that are offensive. Some even become apologetic after being told what they have said is hurtful. Everything is taken concretely and literally. Humor may be very difficult if not impossible for them to grasp. Some require constant prompting. These problems make normal social interaction very difficult. These disturbances may result in secondary social avoidance because of the severe inability to read and understand social cues. These individuals lack what might appear to them as a sixth sense which non-autistic individuals seem to possess. Children in both categories often have varying degrees of poor or inadequate eye contact. As mentioned earlier, the presence of poor eye contact is not necessarily a result of avoiding another person's face or eyes, but may be a severe impairment in the individual's attention span, such that just as much time may be spent looking at someone's face or eyes as the surrounding objects. On top of that, eye-to-eye gaze may not be used to communicate nonverbally as is done by non-autistic individuals.

Although children with autism have a variety of social and cognitive deficits, they also possess many gifts and talents. Just as a blind person may be compensated with over-development of non-visual senses, individuals with autism may use particular portions of their brain better than most. Many autistic children enjoy memorizing things, and are even able to develop and use algorithms that allow them to make sense of the world. That may explain how a young child may be able to determine a particular date or day of the week far in advance, the so-called calendar memory. Many autistic children may have an excellent, sometimes photographic memory. There are autistic savants also. A perfect example is Kim Peek who the character in Rain-man was based upon. NASA scientists are trying to understand his brain. Although he is delayed in some areas (he does not know how to dress himself), he has been able to memorize 7,600 books and every zip code, highway and television station in the US. He has also been found to have genius abilities in the fields of history, literature, geography, music and several other areas.

Key Points

- The autistic mind has characteristic strengths as well as weaknesses.

- Individuals with autism are set in their ways mentally they therefore require frequent prompting when new situations arise.

- Psychogenic disturbances play a larger role in autism.

- Social interaction deficit is perhaps the central abnormality in autism.

- The autistic mind is influenced by intrinsic as well as extrinsic factors.

7

BEHAVIOR AND AUTISM

- Why are there so many negative behavioral disturbances in autism?

- Behaviors in autism are bad from whose perspective?

- Are there good behaviors germane to autism?

- What biological factors affect behavior in autism?

- What can we learn about behavior from autism?

The set of symptoms that cause the most dismay to parents are the behavioral disturbances affecting children with autism. This is what leads many parents and doctors to start on the path of pharmaceutical intervention with all types of drugs such as antipsychotics, antidepressants and anxiolytics. The behavior can cause parents to develop stress and anxiety symptoms themselves. This is very important because autistic children often will feed on the parents' anxiety and a vicious interactive cycle begins. Parental anxiety and despair is part of the illness process that complicates autism, although it is hard to avoid.

The cause of behavioral problems must be completely investigated and understood. Therapy and treatment options that simply suppress or cover-up symptoms are not useful and may eventually backfire. Behavioral dysfunction is a result of cognitive deficits, stress, frustration, and mood disturbances. To understand this, consider what would happen to you if you suddenly became blind through no fault of your own. Your behavior would change. Your mood would eventually be affected, which would further affect your behavior. In the case of autism, it is a bit more complicated. Imagine a child who does not know that he has an auditory processing deficit. What he hears is significantly distorted. He cannot understand, and does not know why he cannot understand. He gets frustrated. It gets worse because outsiders may not know that this child, who may

57

have normal intelligence and has passed a couple of hearing tests, is not able to comprehend their words. This causes the child's behavior to continue to spiral downward. An adult with autism once described to me how frustrating it was for him as a nonverbal child. Even though with therapies he had improved in several areas, he was still nonverbal. He could speak in his mind but simply could not figure out how to get the words out. This was very frustrating. Fortunately, he later became verbal and now has excellent, articulate speech.

Apart from psychosocial causes, behavioral disturbances such as tantrums may result from biological problems. The following are examples of biological dysfunctions that likely affect many children's behavior with autism:

- Gastrointestinal abnormalities

  - Most commonly gastroesophageal reflux causing discomfort

  - Esophagitis (for example yeast related)

  - Stomachache from a variety of sources

- Headaches

  - Most typically migraine headaches

  - Headaches from other sources such as:

    - Seizures

    - Food allergies/intolerances

    - Toxic/metabolic dysfunction

- Sensory processing problems, especially painful hearing

With respect to behavior and autism, the term 'bad' may be a relative term. I have seen many cases where a behavior that was labeled bad was found to be not only involuntary but one that was predicated on a treatable though unidentified problem. Unfortunately, the behavioral problems may have a component of strong defiance that may be hard to deal with, but may be related to a specific underlying disturbance. The overwhelming majority of children with autism are strongwilled. This may be a defensive mechanism to help the child cope with the underlying problems present. Thus, a child who refuses to break away from a routine may simply be protecting himself from the unknown, and subconsciously guarding himself from a situation that brings discomfort. Bad behavior then may actually be better defined as coping behaviors that to others appear 'horrible'. Understood this way, outsiders should view autistic children with annoying behaviors with compassion and understanding. Before attempting to extinguish a 'bad' behavior, it is important to try to understand the source or etiology of the behavior, and remove the reason for the behavior if possible.

Despite what I mentioned above, it should be noted that children with autism can also engage in bad behavior of which they are fully conscious and for which they should be disciplined appropriately. The important issue however is to try to distinguish, as in other areas the 'WONT" and "CANT". This important question is discussed in more detail in Chapter 23.

<u>Key Points</u>

- Behavioral problems in autism may be the most difficult to deal with.

- Behavioral problems may be triggered by psychological, social, or biological factors.

- Behavioral problems can best be treated by acknowledging the underlying cause.

- Hyperacusis (sensitivity to sound) is a common cause of behavioral disturbances.

- It is always important to distinguish between "won't" and "can't" or non compliance versus inability.

8

THE GENETICS OF AUTISM

- What role do genes and heredity play in autism?

- Are the sex chromosomes affected?

- How many genes are affected in autism?

- What is the relationship between genetic defect and metabolic abnormality?

- How do genetic factors relate to environmental ones?

With the completion of the human genome project we now have a comprehensive view of our genetic legacy. In the case of autism and other neuropsychiatric conditions, however, the task of understanding the role of genes remains tricky and challenging. Neuropsychiatric conditions are not generally explained by a single gene defect. Not only must we look for the various genes that may be playing a role in these disorders, we must also try to understand how genes interact with environmental factors. But is autism really genetically based? How can we answer that question?

When autism affects one identical twin, it affects the other 75 % of the time. The concordance rate for fraternal twins, however, is only approximately 3%. The sibling risk rate is between 2.8%-7.0%. Autism-related symptoms occur in up to 20% of siblings. It is interesting to note the biopsychosocial profile of many individuals with autism. This was first noted and mentioned by Leo Kanner himself. The 11 children he evaluated had parents that in his words were "highly intelligent". These parents were successful. Interestingly, regarding the fathers he reported (he wrote this in 1943):

- Four children had fathers that were psychiatrists.

- One had a father that was "a brilliant lawyer".

- One father was a chemist and law school graduate.

- One father was a plant pathologist.

- Another father was a professor of forestry.

- One father had a degree in law and studied at three universities.

- One father was a mining engineer.

- One father was a successful businessman.

Regarding the mothers Kanner reported:

- Nine of the eleven mothers were college graduates.

- One was a freelance writer.

- One was a psychologist.

- One was a physician.

- One was a graduate nurse.

Kanner went on to report that many of the grandparents and relatives of the children were scientists, physicians, writers, journalists and students of art. He also stated "all but three of the families are represented either in the Who's Who in America or in American Men of Science or in both". In my personal experience, I have also found the above to be true for a significant proportion of my patients. Many of the parents have advanced degrees or are very successful.

The field of behavioral genetics suggests that not just one gene influences behavior, rather there are multiple genes involved. Since 1996, there has been an international collaborative effort to identify the specific genes influencing autism. The Autism Genetics Cooperative is a group of researchers and clinicians working with the help of families with children affected by autism to find the genetic cause(s). New genetic models for explaining autism have emerged include the MEGDI (mixed epigenetic and genetic and mixed de novo and inherited) model. According to this model, there is an epigenetic as well as genetic explanation that results in autism. Instead of a problem with gene sequence there can also be a problem with gene expression from genomic imprinting where maternal versus paternal transmission of a gene can alter genetic expression in a specific way. De novo disturbances can also arise.

The main chromosomal abnormalities that are being looked at today include problems with the following five chromosomes:

- Chromosome 2 (genes involved in gastrointestinal function)

- Chromosome 3 (genes involved in early brain development and GABA function)

- Chromosome 7 (gene for regulation and formation of brain cells)

- Chromosome 15 (same gene involved in Angelman syndrome and one that is associated with GABA receptors. There is also a protein which regulates ions)

- Chromosome X (genes involved in social skills and nerve cell interaction)

Regarding the X chromosome, one condition that should be highlighted is Fragile X. Fragile X is the leading inherited cause of mental retardation. It is a relatively common genetic cause of autism as well. It is interesting to note the variation in clinical presentation of this condition. It ranges from mild learning disabilities to severe autism. There are several neuropsychiatric disturbances in Fragile X including, anxiety, OCD, tactile defensiveness and in some cases seizures. Physical features include: high arched palate, lazy eye, large ears, flat feet and low muscle tone. Apart from Fragile X syndrome, various other genetic and chromosomal problems have been reported as mentioned below.

GENETIC AND CHROMOSOMAL PROBLEMS ASSOCIATED WITH AUTISM:

Del 1q43, del 15q, interstitial del 17 (p11.2), t (1; 7; 21), 3p-, 5p+, 8p-, 17p-, 18q-,

t(5;6) (q13;p23), t(3;12) (p26.3;q23.3), t(X;8) (p22.13;q22.1), t(22,13), t(1;15) (p35;q1233),

Trisomy 21, trisomy 22, partial trisomy 16p,

Iso Y dup q11-21, inv Y (p11; q11), iso Y dup q11-21,

Monosomy (5 pter-5p15.3),

XXX, XXY, XYY, XXYY, Large Y,

Adrenomyloneuropathy, Angelman's syndrome, Basal cell nevus syndrome, Ceroid storage disease, Cohen syndrome, Cornelia de Lange Syndrome, Duchene's muscular dystrophy, Fragile X syndrome, Goldenhar's syndrome, Histidinemia, Hurler's syndrome, Hypomelanosis of Ito, Joubert's syndrome, Mobius syndrome, Neurofibromatosis, Neurolipodisis, Noonan's syndrome, Oculocutaneous albinism, Peter's Plus syndrome, Phenylketonuria (untreated), Sanfilippo's syndrome, type A, Shprintzen's syndrome, Marshall-Smith syndrome, Tuberous Sclerosis, Williams syndrome and XLMR with Marfanoid habitus (from the Textbook of Pediatric Neuropsychiatry).

Like other fields of research in autism, genetics is very active and hopeful. This information can only be useful clinically though if the genetic abnormalities found can explain the 'how' of autism symptoms. There needs to specifically be an understanding of how the genetic abnormalities relate to metabolic problems. In the case of fragile X, for instance, researchers have been able to demonstrate how a single gene mutation can affect a protein called FMRP (fragile X retardation protein). Without this protein, there is dysregulation of brain cells as they are unable to communicate with each other properly. This leads to the variety of problems seen in people affected with fragile X syndrome. This sort of information is very useful.

In other individuals with autism, we know that genes play a strong role, but multiple genes are likely involved. For now, we must use the information available to us including detailed family histories, close examination of perinatal factors, associated morbidities, and attribute the rest to environmental factors.

Key Points

- Genes play a vital role in the development of autism.

- There are a variety of genetic disorders that are associated with autism.

- In most cases of autism, there may be several genes involved.

- Fragile X is the most common genetic disorder associated with autism.

• The practical implication of genetic defects in autism is their toxic-metabolic correlate.

9

THE DAN! MODEL OF AUTISM

- What is DAN?

- How did DAN! get started?

- What is the importance of DAN!

- How can you find a DAN! Doctor?

- Are their any concerns with the DAN! movement?

Dr. Bernard Rimland, the research psychologist who was instrumental in dismantling Bettelheim's psychogenic theory of autism, has supported the notion that autism should be thought of as a biologically treatable condition. Dr. Rimland has in fact started a very important movement called DAN! This stands for Defeat Autism Now! The main objective is to do just that, i.e. Defeat Autism Now! Dr. Rimland, who also started the Autism Society of America, has played a historical role in the evolution of autism's history (see Chapter 1). At this time autism is gaining more recognition, and more individuals are being diagnosed. Many theories have emerged as to why the incidence of the disorder has increased, and the research is ongoing.

As a health conscious physician, I have always valued the role of good nutrition in health and the prevention of illness. I have also been aware of the connection between the function of the neurologic, gastrointestinal and immunologic systems. DAN doctors and researchers, in general understand the importance of nutritional and environmental factors in autism.

The DAN movement is comprised of a group of doctors, clinicians and researchers who understand and are devoted to the treatment and eradication of autism. DAN practitioners are usually good listeners, open-minded, and understand the concerns pertaining to nutrition, vaccination, and other environmental factors. Because this movement is so important and many families are trying to implement DAN protocols, and because waiting lists to see DAN practitioners may be long, I will explain certain DAN ideas as I see them. We always encourage families to seek professional help, but there are certain things that can be done *safely* before you visit a DAN practitioner, if you choose to see a DAN! doctor.

The DAN philosophy can simply and succinctly be summarized like this:

An infant comes into this world with some genetic vulnerability (immune, metabolic, or toxic). After an environmental exposure, such as with vaccines or Thimerosal a susceptible infant becomes injured. This injury may be compounded by multiple rounds of broad spectrum antibiotics that are prescribed for the child, who seems to have a weakened or disturbed immune system. These antibiotics destroy the balance between good (probiotics) and bad bacteria (pathogens), such that there is an overgrowth of yeast leading to a condition called *gut dysbiosis*. Due to yeast there is a release of various toxins that impair gut activity contributing to the so-called *leaky gut syndrome*. Neurological function is impaired as a result of the release of neurotoxins. The impaired integrity of the gut wall, allows various macromolecules (improperly digested food substances), toxins, and pathogens to pass through the gut wall and into the circulation. This puts a strain on the liver which has to work harder to detoxify these foreign substances. Food allergies or sensitivities develop because the immune system becomes overactive. This further impairs the integrity of the gut wall. As the immune system becomes weaker, the child falls prey to more infections with more antibiotics being prescribed. This leads to a vicious cycle. Due to oral defensiveness with various textures of food, reflux and other related-problems, eating habits become poor and this leads to malnourishment. The malnourishment is also due to metabolic disturbances that are innate to the child. Metabolic derangements in various detoxification systems and the inability to break down casein and gluten (found in dairy and wheat respectively) guarantee an endogenous state of intoxication accounting for many of the symptoms noted in the autistic child. You then have a child who has a broken immune, nervous and gastrointestinal system.

Based on the above, treatment of autism entails the following:

Fix the gut.
Boost immune function.
Avoid foods that cannot be digested properly (such as gluten and casein)
Avoid all known or suspected food allergens
Nourish the malnourished child with appropriate supplements.
Detoxification using chelation.

A list of the supplements often used:

-TMG (trimethylglycine)/DMG (dimethylglycine)

These are very safe substances considered to be food although they resemble B vitamins. TMG is DMG with an additional methyl group. Many children with autism have shown improvements with DMG and TMG, a food substance first discovered in Russia. DMG and TMG also have a positive affect on the immune system and possibly on seizures.

-B6 (high doses) with magnesium

The effects of B6 and magnesium are well studied. Various studies done in the United States and abroad (Europe) have been positive. Several multivitamins designed for children with ASD have large amounts of B6 and magnesium.

-Digestive enzymes:

These allow for the complete breakdown of allergenic food substances. In children with ASD, it is not unusual to see sensitivities to more than 20 food items. Dairy and wheat products are often included in the list. Some enzymes also allow breakdown of substances known as phenols that many children may not tolerate well.

-Colostrum.

This 'nature's food' is a potent natural immune agent that fights yeast and harmful bacteria while providing the right balance of vitamins, minerals, immune and growth factors.

-Anti-oxidants.

They inhibit cellular damage caused by the action of free radicals. Many anti-oxidants also protect against heavy metal toxicity:

> Coenzyme Q10
> Glutathione (oral, intravenous, or transdermal)
> Selenium and Vitamin E
> Melatonin

-Lauricidin (monolaurin)

This fatty acid substance is very effective and safe. It kills yeast/fungi, bacteria and viruses.

-Cod Liver Oil

Contains both essential fatty acids and vitamin A. There appears to be a subset of children with a G-alpha protein defect who are at risk for the development of autistic symptoms when exposed to the pertussis toxin in the DPT vaccine. These children may do particularly well with a combination of Cod Liver Oil and Urocholine.

-Carnosine (CARN-AWARE):

This is a di-peptide containing two amino acids, histidine and alanine. Dr. Michael Chez, a pediatric neurologist from Illinois, has conducted a double blind placebo controlled study with this naturally occurring substance and found it to be very helpful for several of the symptoms of autism, including expressive and receptive language. An open labeled study showed significant seizure reduction in some children that had failed standard anti-epileptic medication. For further information go to www.car-Aware.com.

-Other amino acid related products

GABA—Several anti-epileptic drugs work on GABA receptors in the brain.
GLUTAMINE—This helps with immune, gut and brain functions.
TAURINE AND GLYCINE—These substances are abundant in the brain. Taurine is so abundant and so vital neurologically that it has been labeled a 'brain amino acid'.

If yeast overgrowth is present, anti-fungal agents can be used

Natural-nonprescription antifungal agents:

Caprylic Acid
Undecylenic Acid
Citrus Extract
Oil of Oregano
Garlic

Prescription antifungal medications

Nystatin—safest
Fluconazole
Ketoconazole
Itraconazole
Terbinafine

Probiotics—These are agents that supply friendly bacteria to the gut, which allows yeast to be kept under good control thereby promoting gut healing. There are many products available at health food stores and other specialized stores. Many include various strains of:

Acidophilus
Lactobacillus

DAN practitioners commonly do certain tests to aid in the treatment of commonly found biochemical abnormalities.

Biomedical testing

The following tests are common examples of tests done to guide biologically based interventions:

Serum Food Allergy Panel—This is a blood test that can detect *IGG*-related food sensitivities that can cause a variety of *delayed* reactions. Depending on the lab used, this test can detect over 100 different food substances that are suspected of causing allergy problems.

Urine Peptides—This test provides evidence of partially degraded particles of gluten and casein. This can indicate if an individual may not be able to tolerate wheat and/or dairy products and that a trial of gluten/casein-free diet is warranted.

Microbial Organic Acid Test—There are certain labs that look for evidence of microbial (yeast) byproducts in addition to the conventional organic acids in the urine. This may be the only way in some individuals to suggest the presence of an intestinal yeast problem we call *gut dysbiosis.*

Comprehensive Digestive Stool Analysis—This test looks at the various abnormalities that may be found in the gut ranging from yeast overgrowth (and other pathogens) to intestinal permeability dysfunction, the so called *leaky gut syndrome.*

Heavy metals—There are several ways of measuring the levels of various toxic heavy metals (e.g. mercury, cadmium, etc.) in the body such as hair, blood, or urine samples. The most accurate way of measuring heavy metals in the body is by using a chelator (a special substance that has the ability to bind metal and cause its excretion from the body). Some heavy metals like mercury may leave the blood stream and reside in various tissues in the body, therefore using a chelator is important. Some blood tests may reveal abnormalities attributable to heavy metal toxic injury.

> **Copper, Zinc, Ceruloplasmin and Metallothionein**—These levels and a ratio between copper/zinc can allow the determination of whether a special protein known as metallothionein is deficient or impaired. This protein malfunctions in many children with ASD and can be treated to a certain extent with appropriate zinc and specific amino acid supplementation.
>
> **Essential Fatty acids**—This is a blood test that is important in ASD children who are picky eaters and those with mood disorders, hyperactivity and short attention span.
>
> **Brain autoimmune panel**—There are specialized labs that measure brain auto-antibodies.

With respect to labs, it is crucial to understand the relationship between an abnormal lab and a clinical manifestation. If, for instance, a yeast problem or casein sensitivity problem is strongly suspected but cannot be substantiated by laboratory findings, the practitioner should still treat the patient accordingly. If there is a positive response to your treatment, your empirical trial becomes the best evidence that there was a problem present. Likewise, an abnormal test does not always translate into a clinical problem. Remember, treat the patient.

The DAN movement has provided a lot of hope for families looking for answers and safe treatment options. This movement is devoted to the unraveling of the biomedical and environmental factors significant in children with ASD. This movement allies itself with and empowers parents who otherwise feel hopeless, helpless, and discouraged.

As with every movement, there are some potential dangers. It is possible under the guise of DAN! for some clinicians to introduce concepts that are pseudoscientific. DAN! practitioners should resist the urge to practice 'cookbook' medicine by prescribing the same type of treatment for every child with autism. Not everyone, for instance, may need to be placed on a GFCF diet. Not everyone may require chelation. The underlying etiology varies for each child. Labs must be interpreted with caution since there is sometimes a tendency to treat the lab instead of the patient. This is particularly important since the specialized labs ordered may be very expensive. Finally, sometimes there seems to be an overemphasis on biomedical or biological disturbances. Broader issues that are non-biological should be incorporated more fully in the DAN! approach to treatment. If this is not done, the DAN! movement runs the risk of becoming as reductionistic as conventional medicine.

Key Points

- According to DAN! autism can be defeated by early identification and treatment.

- Acknowledge the presence of gastrointestinal, immune and brain disturbances.

- First treat the gut. Get rid of yeast.

- When necessary avoid gluten and casein which may not be properly digested.

- Strengthen the immune system.

- Feed the body with appropriate nutrients.

- Remove toxins including heavy metal toxins using chelation.

10

AUTISM AND NEUROPSYCHIATRY

- What does autism teach us about the borderland of psychiatry and neurology?

- Is autism more neurological or psychiatric?

- How significant are non-neuropsychiatric factors in autism?

- Why does the field of autism engender so much controversy?

- Can an understanding of autism help us better understand neuropsychiatry?

1 out of every 6 children in America suffers from problems such as autism, ADHD, dyslexia and aggression
(*US. News & World Report,* June 19, 2000, p.47)

Whether you are a parent of a child with autism, Tourette's syndrome, ADHD, OCD, epilepsy or another neurological/neurobehavioral disorder, it is important to understand the importance of autism. If you are a physician (particularly a neurologist, psychiatrist or developmental pediatrician) or other health professional interested in neurobehavioral disorders, or if you are a therapist, nutritionist or epidemiologist, autism should be of interest to you. Why? Autism is the best example of a disorder that combines neurological, psychogenic, behavioral, emotional, immune, metabolic as well as nutritional disturbances. Some clinicians believe that autism is simply a genetically-based, chronic developmental disorder with its onset in early childhood. Autism is much more than that. Autism is an intricate and multifactorial condition. There is reason to believe that in many cases autism is partly iatrogenic, acquired, and environmentally-based in origin.

An important interface exists between the mind and body and between neurological and psychiatric ailments. Children with autism have both gifts and limitations that require us to redefine our current understanding of the mind and neurological function. Some of the gifts include: *calendar memory* where an individual can name the day of the week that corresponds to any date, even years in advance. Some individuals are *human calculators* and can add or multiply any number in their head. Some have perfect pitch. On occasion, an autistic individual diagnosed with severe mental retardation may be able to play music by ear, even complicated musical pieces after only hearing the music piece once. Other gifts include: photographic memory and artistic talents. Many children with autism are unusually sensitive to things that do not affect others like weather, changes in routine, sounds, and fluorescent lights, to list a few. Many children with autism, on the other hand may have decreased reactivity to pain and certain auditory stimuli. This suggests that certain portions of the brain are turned on 'high' perception, while other portions are turned down 'low'. Those portions of the brain which are tuned to low perception may be a form of defense mechanism for the child.

Autism is a medical condition that stimulates controversy. This is partly because it cannot be diagnosed with a laboratory test. Conditions like autism, which cannot be diagnosed with a laboratory test can lead to disputes with respect to their cause, treatment, and etiology. In the case of autism, there is a large division. Some believe in a biomedical paradigm that can explain the etiology of autism and whereby biological interventions can be used to treat and sometimes reverse autism. These paradigms look at nutrition and environmental factors, such as vaccines and toxic heavy metals, as playing an important causative role in autism. Conversely, there are others that believe that vaccines, heavy metals, and nutrition have little or nothing to do with autism. Autism is a genetic developmental condition. It is viewed as a brain disorder which requires pharmacological intervention in palliating symptoms in what is considered a life-long disorder. Reports of 'an autism epidemic' are viewed with great skepticism. Alternative explanations for the increase in the incidence of autism are offered such as better diagnosing techniques, revised diagnostic criteria, and greater awareness of the problem. Parents of children with autism are caught in the middle of the controversy, and are often overwhelmed by the conflicting information available. The problem is compounded by the varied treatment and therapeutic options available. They are purported to be life-saving but are they genuine or not. How can you tell the difference?

Autism is a disorder with diverse symptoms. In addition to the core diagnostic deficits, many children with autism have seizures, sensory processing disturbances, obsessive compulsive disorder, attention deficit hyperactivity disorder, tic disorders, mood disorders, anxiety disorders, immune disturbances, and gastrointestinal dysfunctions. Despite all of these problems, children with autism usually appear normal physically, and routine imaging of the brain is often unremarkable. The lack of objective and universal laboratory finding in diagnosing autism has led to some confusion in the classification of this disorder. Is autism a psychiatric, psychological, psychogenic, behavioral or neurological condition? I believe that all of the above apply. In fact, the one concept that best summarizes autism is **dysregulation**. Autism is a pervasive condition caused by dysregulation leading to impairment of multiple systems of the body. As a result, individuals with autism have a particular neurocircuitry that explains their behavioral and cognitive makeup. Many autistic individuals have immune disturbances or outright autoimmune disorders that undoubtedly relate to the main regulatory abnormalities present. This dysregulation accounts for vulnerabilities that are not only biological but also psychological. Any approach that fails to take into account the multifaceted nature of autism and related conditions is inadequate.

Like autism, most conditions that lie in the borderland of psychiatry and neurology also involve varying levels of dysregulation. Hence, in the case of ADHD, there is a primary dysfunction in regulating sensory input. Trivial and irrelevant stimuli cause distractibility and inability to attend properly. In Tourette's syndrome, there is failure to properly regulate motor movements and impulses leading to tics. With OCD, intrusive thoughts and acts occur due to dysregulation. With bipolar disorder, mood is improperly regulated. Understanding the factors that lead to dysregulation and how to restore regulation is paramount. This understanding not only can allow a better understanding of how to approach neuropsychiatric problems in general, but it also elucidates important factors pertaining to mental and neuronal function.

The mind affects brain activity just as much as neuronal activity determines mental function. Psychosomatic interactions when impaired due to regulatory abnormalities can lead to conditions that take their toll on both mental and somatic functions. By studying autism, we are really exploring the interface between the mind and the brain, nature and nurture, and the human experience in general.

Key Points

- Autism is perhaps the most fascinating, complex, intriguing and controversial neuropsychiatric disorder.

- Dysregulation is the one concept that best summarizes the etiology of autism and the basis for its clinical manifestations.

- Like autism, most neuropsychiatric conditions involve some form of dysregulation which explains the primary underlying disturbance.

- A serious study of autism allows a deeper understanding of the properties of the human mind, brain function and psychosomatic interactions.

- Autism can be viewed as a microcosm that reflects the complexities, controversies and diversity of neuropsychiatric ailments in general.

PART II

EVALUATION OF AUTISM

11

RECOGNIZING THE FIRST SIGNS OF AUTISM

- What are the earliest signs of autism?

- How soon can one start the evaluation process?

- How early can a child be diagnosed with autism?

- Are there any prenatal clues?

- What is the importance of detecting early signs?

Any child suspected of having autism should be evaluated expediently. In some cases an evaluation may reveal that the child has delays that are mild and fall outside of the spectrum of autism. Then there will be situations where the diagnosis will fit the definition of ASD. In any case an evaluation is necessary to make that determination. According to the National Institutes of Health and the U.S. Department of Education, early screenings of children for ASD should be encouraged. The following are early clues that should alert observers to the possibility of autism in a young child:

- **Social Concerns**

  Seems to prefer to play alone
  Has poor eye contact
  Is in his/her own world
  Is not interested in other children
  Does not smile socially
  Lack of pretend play
  Lack of social play
  Lack of declarative pointing (pointing for shared attention)

Lack of gaze monitoring (turning to look in the same direction as an adult)
Lack of joint attention

• **Behavioral Concerns**

Tantrums
Lines things up
Is oversensitive to certain textures or sounds
Has unusual attachment to selected toys
Gets stuck on things over and over

• **Communication Concerns**

Does not respond to his/her name
Cannot tell you what s/he wants
Appears deaf at times
Does not point or wave bye-bye
Does not follow directions
Used to say a few words but now does not

CONCERNS THAT WARRANT IMMEDIATE EVALUATION

No babbling by 12 months
No gesturing (pointing, waving bye-bye, etc.) by 12 months
No single words by 16 months
No 2-word spontaneous phrases by 24 months
ANY loss of ANY language or social skills at ANY age

It has been noted by some experts that by four months of age, infants should make anticipatory motor adjustment. For example, when an infant is picked up an anticipatory motor adjustment would be facial tension and shoulder shrugging. In the case of autism, this may not occur until much later in development. This failure of anticipatory motor adjustment may be an early clue to the possibility of a child having autism.

Another interesting finding is that many children with autism have large heads, or what is known as macrocephaly. Interestingly, Leo Kanner first made this observation in 5 of his 11 patients. This relative enlargement of the head is related to brain enlargement. The head size of many children with autism is actually on the smaller side at birth but then there is accelerated head growth leading to a larger than normal head size in the first few years of life. By adolescence or early adulthood, the head size is no longer larger than normal. This early increase in head size may be the earliest sign suggestive of autism. As with seizures, this is evidence that autism is a neurological disorder. The increased head size is secondary to megalencephaly (increased brain size). Both the white and gray matter of the cerebrum is increased and the amount of white matter is increased in the cerebellum based on radiographic studies.

The importance of early recognition is for early intervention to be made on behalf of children with neuropsychiatric disorders. This does not mean that an older autistic child or adult cannot improve significantly with treatment initiated later in life. Neuroscientists have recently discovered that adult mice were able to develop new brain pathways. The brains or the rats were rewired to receive visual cues in the hearing part of their brains. This study, conducted at MIT (MIT Tech Talk Volume 44, number 1; 9/1/04) led to the conclusion that: "adult brains show more plasticity than previously believed".

Key Points

- Early suspicion of autism is crucial for the early initiation of treatment. The earlier treatment is initiated, the better.

- Lack of declarative pointing may be one of the earliest social deficits seen in autism.

- Children with autism may initially appear deaf. They may not respond when their name is called.

- The earliest physical sign of autism may be the presence of a larger than normal increase in head size.

- Although treatment should start as early as possible, even adults may show significant improvement with appropriate interventions.

12

THE ROLE OF PARENTS IN THE EVALUATION PROCESS

- Why should parents play a major role in the evaluation of autism?

- How can parents become better evaluators?

- How soon should the evaluation start?

- What can distract parents from a good evaluation process?

- What are the rewards of a good evaluation?

The medical history is very important in the evaluation of autism. Parents should be ready to provide the following information to their evaluator:

- Onset of noticeable symptoms
  - Were abnormalities noted from birth?
  - Did the child seem normal then regress?
  - When did regression occur?
    - Did any event seem to precede the regression?
- Presence of perinatal abnormalities (e.g. hypoxia, neonatal infection/fever)
- Neurological symptoms
  - Activity suggestive of seizures (see Appendix F)
  - Coordination difficulties
  - Progressive cognitive decline

- This may suggest a degenerative neurometabolic condition
- Tone abnormalities
  - Hypotonia (low muscle tone)
  - Spasticity or hypertonia (muscle stiffness)
- Sensory abnormalities
  - Poor vision (or light sensitivity)
  - Poor hearing
  - Hyperacusis
- Family history and profile
  - Family history of ASD
  - Family history neurobehavioral abnormalities (e.g. Tourette's syndrome)
  - Family history of autoimmune disease (.e.g. lupus, multiple sclerosis, etc.)
  - Family history of mood disorder (depression or bipolar disorder)
  - Family history of anxiety disorder (e.g. OCD)
  - Family history of personality traits (introversion/extroversion/obsession)

Never take anything for granted. Each piece of information may be useful though it may seem trivial. In my practice I have had several parents relate 'by the way' information at the end of the visit that turned out to be very important. In some cases I was able to obtain valuable information only after the second or third visit. For example, if your child has an unexplained exacerbation of annoying self-stimulatory behavior:

- Carefully document the self-stimulatory behavior including anything that the child ate, drank, infections/fever that precipitated the events, any drugs, or supplements that are related to the event. Although natural supplements are safe, some may not be the right ones for your child. Also make note of any environmental changes, as well as psychosocial stressors the child experiences.

- Remove any perceived stresses or triggers from the child's environment.

- It is important for the parents themselves not to be stressed since the child can feed on the parents' stress, which can further aggravate the self-stimulatory behaviors. At times it may mean that the parents need to completely ignore the self-stimulatory behaviors. Unlike some forms of epileptic motor seizures that can be harmful if they persist for more than several minutes, this is not the case with self-stimulatory behaviors. They may be annoying, they may appear bizarre, you may want to remove them, but the fact is that they do not harm the brain. That means there is time to patiently work at removing the stressors that cause the behaviors.

• It is of vital importance to make sure that the child's diet is healthy, well-balanced, and well supplemented with the appropriate nutrients. Often, that alone can completely eliminate the self-stimulatory behaviors. Metabolic issues, detoxification problems, and infections (bacterial and fungal/yeast) can trigger tics, and should be appropriately identified and treated.

• Know your child's mode of learning and be aware of any sensory processing difficulties that are present. For instance, if your child has a sound sensitivity, or what is commonly referred to as painful hearing, it is possible in that the self-stimulatory behaviors may be the result of over exposure to certain harmful sounds. The same can apply for visual sensory disturbances.

Since some self-stimulatory behaviors may be comforting mechanisms, it only makes sense that before you try to extinguish a particular behavior you find a replacement behavior that is also soothing.

Key Points

• Parents play a vital role in the early recognition, treatment, support and advocacy of a child with autism.

• Parents should always pay close attention to details, documenting important symptoms of their child. They should act as *medical detectives.*

• Parents must interface well with their child, clinicians, and others in general.

• Parents should recognize that their strength is the child's strength, their stress is the child's stress, their optimism and hope is the child's security and self-confidence.

• Parents should always be hopeful, and never give-up.

13

TACKLING AUTISM USING A TEAM APPROACH

- Why is a team approach important?

- Who should be part of the team?

- How can you make sure you have the best team for your child?

- What role should parents play in the team?

- Who should be the coordinator of the team?

Team members

PHYSICIANS

Primary care physician
Pediatric Neurologist
Child Psychiatrist
Developmental Pediatrician
Other specialists depending on the case

    Gastroenterologist
    Immunologist
    Endocrinologist
    Geneticist

PSYCHOLOGISTS

General psychologist
Neuropsychologist

THERAPISTS

Speech/language therapist
Occupational therapist (preferably one trained in sensory integration therapy)
Behavioral therapist/consultant
Physical therapist

EDUCATIONAL SPECIALISTS (Especially those with experience in autism)

Finding the right team members may be difficult. All the team members should be competent, caring, understanding and have the ability to communicate with the other team members. It is very important that all team members be on the same wavelength in terms of optimism and enthusiasm for success. A professional team can be very valuable in analyzing a given problem or set of problems from various angles. Bringing different expertise to the table can allow a problem to be solved efficiently even if it is complex. Each team member serves a different function, but all the members are important. The coordinator should be one who can interpret all the test results, and assess overall progress. Ideally, the coordinator should be the primary care physician. Of course, parents are the non-medical coordinators of the patient as well.

It is useful for parents to ask as many questions as necessary from each team member so that they clearly understand the treatment plan. If a child is not progressing with a given treatment plan, the plan needs to be re-evaluated and possibly changed. Each clinic visit should have a purpose. There should always be a general game plan. Finding all of the team members may take time. There are always some things that can be started by parents until the team is formed, such as instituting proper nutrition and lifestyle.

Key Points

- A child with autism should be treated by a team of specialized individuals.

- There should be a coordinator.

- Good communication between all team members is necessary.

- There are safe interventions that parents can start on their own such as proper nutrition and lifestyle.

- Various specialists may be needed depending on a child's particular problems.

- It is always ideal to work with individuals that understand and have experience with autism.

14

GENERAL EVALUATION

- What are the components of a general evaluation?

- Who should do the general evaluation?

- Should the same battery of tests be done on every autistic child?

- How often is testing necessary?

- What labs should be used?

GENERAL TESTS

The following may be helpful:

- CBC (complete blood count)

- Iron studies

- Thyroid function tests

- Chemistry profile

- Copper, zinc and lead levels

- Magnesium

More specific investigations are necessary depending on additional problems that may be present for each individual child. Depending on the therapies that are being done, some tests need to be repeated. If a patient is healthy and is doing well, certain tests such as a chemistry profile and CBC should be checked at least once a year.

GENETIC TESTING

- High resolution chromosomes

- Fragile X

If there is a family history of autistic symptoms and/or dysmorphic features are present, a genetics referral should be obtained. In select cases some specific genetic testing (e.g. FISH studies for subtelomeric deletions or other specialized tests) may be warranted.

METABOLIC TESTING

At the very least the following should be considered:

- Serum amino acids

- Urine organic acids

- Serum lactate and pyruvate

- Urine uric acid

- Ammonia

More specialized metabolic tests will be decided upon by your specialist based on the evaluation, such as:

- Carbohydrate deficient transferin

    One should consider the possibility of a glycosylation disorder (i.e. glycoprotein metabolism abnormality). There are various types of glycosylation disorders. Several are associated with immune dysfunction, gastrointestinal disorders, seizures, and speech/language impairment. All of which are reported in autism

- Biotin

- Acylcarnitine profile

- Carnitine

- Very long chain fatty acids

- Uric acid

- Purine/pyrimidine disorders

  Lech-Nyhan Syndrome

Some of the above metabolic tests are screening tests. If abnormal, further testing may be required. There are various other tests that are usually checked by DAN doctors that have already been discussed in Chapter 9.

<u>Key Points</u>

- Routine tests should be part of the evaluation.

- Genetic testing may be helpful in certain patients.

- Metabolic testing may be necessary in some patients.

- The best test in some cases is an empirical trial of a particular therapy.

15

THE NEUROLOGICAL EVALUATION

- What are the components of a neurological evaluation?

- Why is a neurological evaluation essential?

- Who should perform the neurological evaluation?

- Why should the possibility of seizures always be considered?

- Why should sensory function always be assessed?

It is always necessary to have a good general assessment made of the patient. In addition, a detailed neurological examination is required. A neurologist should perform the neurological assessment as they are the most qualified persons to do so. The following should be checked:

- The senses (hearing and vision).

- The possibility of seizures or 'epileptic aphasia'. A neurologist can perform an EEG.

- The skin. Some neurocutaneous disorders are associated with autism such as tuberous sclerosis.

- Dysmorphic features which would suggest a possible chromosomal disorder.

- Tone. Significant hypertonia in the distal lower extremities can indicate static encephalopathy (cerebral palsy). These children may walk on their toes at all times.

NEUROLOGICAL TESTING

- EEG—this is mandatory since seizures are common. Some seizures may be subtle or subclinical. A normal EEG does not necessarily rule out seizures. A child may need a sleep-deprived EEG or even a 24-hour ambulatory EEG.

- NEUROIMAGING—this is necessary when the neurological examination is abnormal or a structural brain abnormality is suspected. The imaging modality of choice is MRI (magnetic resonance imaging). Imaging is not necessary in every case. Apart from an MRI, there are other imaging modalities of the brain including PET and SPECT scans. The former is a radiographic test that utilizes de-oxyglucose to identify abnormal metabolic areas of functioning in the brain. The SPECT scan looks at blood flow to the brain as an indicator of brain dysfunction.

- NEUROMETABOLIC TESTING—a neurologist will do in-depth neurometabolic testing as dictated by the patient's neurologic presentation. Many neurologists will get a basic neurometabolic screen in cases of autism (see Chapter 14).

Key Points

- Always consider the possibility of seizures in a child with autism.

- A normal EEG does not rule out seizures. A sleep deprived or even 24-hour EEG may be required to document seizures.

- Sensory function should always be evaluated.

- When an underlying focal neurological lesion is suspected neuroimaging is always necessary.

- A neurologist should be involved in the care of a child with autism.

16

PSYCHOSOCIAL EVALUATION

- What factors should be considered with a psychosocial evaluation?

- Who should do the evaluation?

- How are social factors important?

- What does a social evaluation entail?

- What are the benefits of a good psychosocial evaluation?

Ideally, every child with autism or another neuropsychiatric condition requires a full psychological assessment. This assessment can provide useful information regarding areas of strengths and weakness. Various areas of cognitive functioning may be explored and deficiencies uncovered, such as learning disorders. This sort of information is invaluable to assist a child in his academic journey. A child's personality traits can be identified also. I use the term *apparent strengths and weaknesses*, because although the tests are well designed and administered by competent specialists, the results may not always reflect the child's true abilities. In particular, tests scores may be lower, sometimes significantly so, than the child's actual level of cognitive ability. There are several reasons for this. A child may not always be able, motivated, or willing to put forth their best effort. The testing may not always be tolerated because its length may be prohibitive. A child may have a correctable impairment such as a sensory disturbance, processing issue, or seizures that may result in a different test score than if the previously mentioned problems were corrected. Children with a known medical or processing problem should have the problem corrected first before testing is obtained, if possible. In many cases, psychological testing may already have been done. If correctable problems are identified after testing has already been obtained then the child should be appropriately treated and retesting should be done for a more accurate reflection of the child's abilities.

No matter how good and detailed the test may be, it still may not reflect a child's full potential, and therefore may not accurately predict the child's prognosis for the future. Psychological testing, as far as I am concerned, should be used as an additional tool in the quest to optimize a child's level of functioning. Even when the test scores are less than desired or expected, this should not be a reason for discouragement or hopelessness.

Apart from psychological evaluations, every child should have a social evaluation. By that I mean that social factors that may play a role in the child's condition should be assessed and addressed. Formal testing with a counselor may be requested to assess the family dynamics. It may be discovered that one parent is better equipped to control the child's behavior than the other, or that one parent's stress affects the child negatively. Apart from the home, social interactions with peers and school personnel should be explored also. Some children with behavioral regression/aggression may be reacting to circumstances at school that are distressing to the child causing stress that is expressed as bad behavior or excessive self-stimulatory behaviors. It is the parents' responsibility to see why and how a particular setting affects the child's behavior. Is there a problem with the structure that is provided to the child? Does the child need more structure of less? Is the environment noisy or distracting? Certain social situations that are minor to a non-autistic individual may present a significant problem for a person with autism. The net effect for the child is the development of stress.

Stress is significant for a child with autism. Children with autism do not handle stress in ways that other people can understand or feel comfortable with. Tantrums, prolonged screaming fits, rage attacks, unusual behaviors, tics, and self-stimulatory behaviors may be a result of stress. Stress affects the mental, emotional, and biological health of people, including children with autism. We are equipped to handle intermittent episodes of stress via the fight or flight response, which temporarily mobilizes catecholamines and prepares the body for unexpected danger. Once the danger is past, the chemicals in the body should return to their baseline level of functioning. With chronic or excessive stress, these biological and chemical changes persist even when the danger or stressor is removed. This eventually leads to behavioral and biological problems for the individual.

Chronic stress, no matter what the cause, is harmful to the body and mind and should therefore be avoided.

There are a variety of rating scales and questionnaires that are used to assess the overall impact of stress upon an individual:

Parenting Stress Index (PSI-III)
Parental Stress Scale (PSS)
Questionnaire on Resources and Stress (QRS)
Family Adaptability and Cohesion Evaluation Scales III (FACES).

When all of the significant psychosocial problems that affect an individual are identified and properly addressed, not only will the person benefit, but so will the family, the caregivers, and everyone involved in the person's care.

Key Points

- A psychological evaluation is always important.

- Social factors should be considered and factored into an autistic child's symptomatology.

- Testing can be done by either a psychologist or neuropsychologist.

- Stress plays a key role in autism.

- There are a variety of questionnaires and rating scales that can help assess the level of stress present and its impact on family interactions

17

EDUCATIONAL NEEDS ASSESSMENT

- Should children with autism be considered disabled?

- What are IEP, IDEA, and section 504?

- What challenges do gifted autistic children experience in school?

- What type of testing in necessary?

- When should educational testing begin?

Children with autism have the potential to learn, but they have greater obstacles to their learning. Children with autism often have to be taught *how* to learn, since this may not come instinctively. Although most children with autism appear normal physically, all autistic children have some degree of cognitive and social limitations, which cause a disability even in those children that are gifted. These children, therefore, require additional assistance with their learning. All children with a suspected or obvious learning difficulty (with or without autism) should have an evaluation to identify any problems that may interfere with their learning. Some learning problems may be more obvious than others. Examples include:

- Basic sensory problem

  - Partial hearing loss

  - Partial visual loss

- Sensory perceptual problem

  - Central auditory processing problem

- With or without hyperacusis
- Visual processing problem
- Specific learning disorder
  - Dyslexia
  - Acalculia
  - Nonverbal learning disorder
- Neurological problems
  - Always rule out seizures
  - Migraine headaches
  - Sleep disturbances
    - These can lead to fatigue, excessive daytime sleepiness, concentration problems and behavioral impairment
  - Movement disorders (especially if excessive or disruptive)
    - Tics
    - Self-stimulatory behaviors
  - Fine motor difficulties
    - An occupational therapy assessment may be necessary
- General health/systemic issues
  - Nutritional status
  - Metabolic disorder
    - Hypoglycemia or other metabolic problems

I will not discuss the appropriateness of one educational system versus another such as private versus public school, or regular versus home school. The important principle is that the proper placement and support is required for the autistic child to do well academically.

Children with autism may be recognized as having a disability. Apart from autism, though, they may have other disabling conditions including: learning disabilities, hearing impairments, visual impairments, deafness, blindness, speech/ language impairments, orthopedic problems, mental retardation, emotional difficulties, traumatic brain injury, or health impairments. Children with disabilities are entitled by law to a free appropriate public education, designed to meet the child's individual educational needs. Children that are gifted are also entitled to the rights that children with disabilities are entitled to. This guarantee of an education geared to meet the specific needs of each child is made possible through the Individuals with Disabilities Education Act (IDEA). Through IDEA, states can receive federal funding to supplement the cost of educating children with disabilities. Before a child is deemed eligible for special education, a complete evaluation of all areas pertaining to the child's suspected area of disability should be conducted. Even if a child is presently mainstreamed in a regular classroom, once a disability is suspected a thorough evaluation may and should be requested. The evaluation must be provided by the school district, free of charge, at a parents' request.

Ideally, children with autism should have a full neuropsychological evaluation. Independent neuropsychological evaluation may provide more information, but this must be obtained independently at the parents' discretion. All children, whether very gifted or significantly impaired, can benefit from neuropsychiatric testing. This testing provides a full picture of the cognitive functions and limitations of a child, and usually detailed recommendations are usually presented that may be useful in structuring the appropriate educational program for the child.

Parents of children with autism should always consider having an IEP (Individualized Educational Program). An IEP is a written statement of the special services that a child with a disability needs in order to be educated properly. Important conditions and features of an IEP include:

- An IEP must include behavior modification programs.

- It must describe any necessary modifications to the child's regular education classes.

- A school district must provide all programs and services contained in an approved IEP.

- The IEP must be reviewed and revised at least once each year to keep up with the child's needs.

- An IEP may state a specific portion of time that a child can spend with non-disabled children.

- An IEP is developed at a meeting where teachers, school personnel and a representative of the school district are in attendance.

I have attended several IEP meetings of my patients. This is unusual for a pediatric neurologist, but I have learned a lot from these meetings and was also able to provide valuable input. According to the federal law, an IEP should be individualized to meet a child's specific needs, and it must be done with the cooperation and consent of the parents. This means that the parents should be well prepared for the child's IEP. I suggest the following preparation prior to attending the IEP meeting:

- Make a list of all of the child's limitations pertaining to learning.

  - This should be based on personal observation and evaluations made by professional assessments.

- Obtaining a letter from your doctor specifically outlining your child's medical condition.

- Provide literature, if available about how your child's medical condition affects their ability to learn.

I believe that many children with autism have strengths that may not always be appreciated. Parents should make sure that a child is being appropriately challenged. Parents should be very active participants in the IEP process. Ask questions freely and make suggestions. It is important that appropriate modifications not just be discussed but be included in the actual IEP. Once they are placed in the IEP they have to be adhered to. Children with disabilities that are not included under IDEA, for example children with physical injuries may still be covered under *Section 504 of the Rehabilitation act of 1973*. Instead of an IEP, a *504 Plan*, which is different but still effective, can be designed. Consider in advance the relative amount of special education versus regular education your child may require. It is always best to write down your suggestions and take these to the meeting to make sure you do not forget anything.

Key points

- The educational needs of every child with autism should be assessed.

- Children with autism are considered to have a handicap, and thus require assistance in school.

- Gifted children also require special services in school.

- There are a variety of biological and sensory disturbances that can affect a child's educational performance.

- An IEP is an official way of determining and implementing services needed in school to succeed academically.

- Parents should be prepared for the IEP since they can provide valuable input.

18

NONCONVENTIONAL TESTING

- What tests or evaluations can be considered non-conventional?

- Is there a role for non-conventional testing?

- What are the criteria for judging the merits of non-conventional tests?

- What are the most commonly used non-conventional tests?

- Are there any risks in non-conventional testing?

After the diagnosis of autism has been established further testing can be done to determine the underlying cause. Conventionally, neurologists may address the possibility of seizures and also look for a metabolic disorder. Neuroimaging may be considered. If suspected, a referral to a geneticist may be initiated to look for a genetic condition. In a nutshell, that is the bulk of the traditional approach. Almost any other testing may be considered non-conventional testing. I subdivide non-conventional testing into two groups: conventional non-conventional testing and non—conventional non-conventional testing.

Conventional non-conventional testing

In this group, conventional testing is done to answer a non-conventional question. What I mean is that a parent may seek a referral to see a gastroenterologist not only to assess a gastrointestinal condition, but to see if it might be tied to the child's autism. In the field of gastroenterology there are a variety of disturbances that may account for symptoms commonly encountered in autistic children including: diarrhea, constipation, gastro-esophageal reflux, malabsorption, leaky gut syndrome, secretin deficiency, gastritis, esophagitis, esophageal candidiasis, and gastrointestinal dysbiosis. The question someone may ask is whether these abnormalities can significantly contribute to the child's core autistic symptoms? Some would say definitely yes, others would say not at all. In my experience the answer depends. There are children who continue to have the clinical symptoms of autism while others seem to show a remarkable improvement and resolution of their autistic symptoms with correction of their gastrointestinal problems. My recommendation, therefore, is to **ALWAYS TREAT THE GUT!** Referral to a gastroenterologist should thus be considered if there is evidence of a gastrointestinal problem or if such as suspicion exists.

Another example is a referral to an immunologist/allergist. Conventional testing for a problem in this area may be sought looking for a connection between the immune system and autism. Food allergies (specifically IGG RAST testing looking for <u>delayed</u> food reactions) for instance, when diagnosed and treated, in some children can lead to significant clinical improvement. The same holds true for other allergic/immune problems. Because correcting immune-related problems can lead to better systemic health and significantly improve core autistic symptoms, my recommendation is to **ALWAYS TREAT IMMUNE PROBLEMS AND BOOST THE IMMUNE SYSTEM!**

Non-conventional non-conventional testing

These sorts of tests are characterized by the following:

• Most regular doctors are unfamiliar with these types of tests and the interpretation of the results.

• They may be called *functional tests.*

• They may need to be done in specialized laboratories.

• They may not be covered by health insurances.

This group of tests range from potentially useful to full-fledged quackery. The following questions should be asked prior to testing:

• Do the benefits obtained by the test justify the cost of the test?

• How is the test going to change or improve the child's management?

- Why is the benefit of one test over another?

- What are the consequences of a positive test?

- What are the consequences of a negative test?

- What is the false positive rate of the test?

- What is the false negative rate of the test?

- Is the test being done for diagnostic purposes or treatment?

I have encountered cases where very expensive, but entirely useless tests were done. The results <u>completely</u> contradicted validated test results, and moreover were based on principles that were clearly erroneous. Prior to obtaining tests, parents should be analytical and ask the above questions. Regardless of the test, one has to be able to show how the results actually relate to a patient's condition. It is important not to simply chase after a laboratory test result if it is not related to a child's medical problem.

<u>Key points</u>

- There are some useful tests that can be obtained to answer non-conventional questions.

- There are some entirely non-conventional tests that may provide useful answers when it comes to autism.

- There are often risks involved when doing non-conventional testing due to the fact that the information may be erroneous or of dubious clinical significance.

- Critical questions should be asked prior to testing especially if the test is very expensive.

- Tests should be done for a specific purpose, and have some impact on the child's overall management.

PART III

COMPREHENSIVE TREATMENT OF AUTISM

19

ORGANIZED TREATMENT STRATEGY

- How useful is an organized treatment strategy?

- What does an organized and comprehensive treatment strategy entail?

- Is there a balance between generalized and individualized treatment?

- How does one differentiate between breakthrough therapies and quackery?

- What should be the ultimate goal of treatment?

Before we discuss treatment strategies, it is of vital importance to first remember that autism is not just one specific condition but a group of disorders with disparate underlying etiologies. There are general non-specific treatments that can be of benefit to all. However, a clinician should try to discover the specific abnormalities that apply to a particular individual.

The big picture for parents and physicians in treating autism should be as follows:

- Start treatment as soon as possible.

- Identify etiological/causative factors as specifically as possible.

- Realize that there are both primary and secondary problems in ASD. One should specifically look for and address the primary problem.

- Give each treatment/therapy ample time to work, but know when to 'call it quits' on a particular treatment option.

- Be a good observer. Document the effect of every treatment whether beneficial or adverse.

- Acknowledge that what works for one child may not necessarily work for another. It may even cause adverse effects. Focus on <u>your</u> child!

- Always have a high index of suspicion for both seizures and sensory processing disorders.

- Strengthen the immune system and make sure the gut is working well.

- Eat properly, avoid all toxic food substances and take appropriate nutritional supplementation.

- Address psychosocial factors.

- Take into account the body's God-given ability to heal itself and the brain's natural course of maturation.

- Place your ultimate trust in God, the ultimate healer.

- Never ever give up and be optimistic always.

OPTIMIZING TREATMENT

1. Initial consideration should always be directed toward correcting any bio-medical or nutritional problems present.

2. Parents should be organized. I recommend making a checklist of the child's symptoms and your goals for recovery. Apart from a 'master' checklist, specialized lists should be made for each problem addressed by each specialist/therapist.

3. Parents should prepare for each clinic visit. Keep a folder with all relevant medical information. Make a list of all questions, concerns, or important observations about your child.

4. Obtain a detailed family history. This may entail interviewing family members. In general, being a good note keeper with respect to your child's progress can be very useful. Speech and language for instance should be monitored carefully. You can obtain a free brochure from the American Speech-Language Hearing Association that can help you track your child's speech, language, and hearing development.

5. Have a medical coordinator, for example your primary care doctor or autism specialist. Assemble a team formed of clinicians, therapists, educational and behavioral specialists, and support personnel. The purpose of the coordinator is to coordinate communication between the various team members.

6. Do not jump on the latest fad autism treatment. This treatment may not benefit *your* child.

7. There should be no hesitation in seeking help from the appropriate specialist for a problem that requires a particular expertise.

8. There are interventions that can be safely begun before a clinical evaluation by an autism specialist is provided. These include proper nutrition, a positive lifestyle change, and avoidance of toxic substances (i.e. food or other chemicals that cause behavioral/cognitive abnormalities).

9. Each clinician should outline a plan of treatment with a clear identified goal. If it is unclear which direction treatment is going, parents should always ask.

10. It should be recognized that although children with autism have special needs, they also have routine problems like other children. This means that not all of an autistic child's problems are necessarily related to autism.

11. There are two main sorts of treatments and interventions in autism. The first type targets the underlying problem and the second type addresses the symptoms. It is important to keep this distinction in mind. For instance, a child may be very aggressive and be placed on an antipsychotic drug to control behavior. While the behavior may improve, the drug is not meant to address the underlying problem. Symptomatic treatment with drugs may be necessary in some cases but this should not replace the need to find and treat the underlying problem.

12. There is more than one way to address a particular problem. Often, the particular treatment option chosen is based on availability, affordability, and safety.

13. Some children with autism have relatively quick and dramatic responses to treatment while others seem refractory to a variety of treatments. The following are common causes of *refractory* symptoms:

   a.   Some patients may actually be on the road to recovery but simply require more time. Patience is important.

   b.   Many parents assume that if a little of something is good, a lot must be better, for example in the case of natural supplements. In all cases, the individual should be given what is needed and not more. It is possible to over do something good and hence slow down the recovery process.

   c.   Simple factors like better hydration with water, normalizing sleep, and making lifestyle changes can result in dramatic improvement in some 'refractory' cases.

   d.   Co-existing medical problems must be identified and treated.

   e.   Effective treatments and interventions may be hindered by negative factors like pessimism, helplessness, and persistent psychosocial stress in the parent(s) or child.

   f.   A sensory processing defect may be overlooked in a child with severe language deficit and behavioral problems.

No matter how tough things may be, parents should NEVER GIVE UP! With proper treatment your child will improve. As parents you have a lot of stress and other difficulties that coexist with having a child with a complex neuropsychiatric disorder like autism. The frustration created should not be directed against the child, although this may seem unavoidable when you are dealing with constant tantrums and behavioral problems. Parents should always try to address and correct their own stress-related problems. I often tell parents to lavish their child with praise and to do so constantly and consistently since children respond to praise.

Someone once wrote the following:

Children Learn What They Live

If a child lives with criticism, he learns to condemn.
If he lives with hostility, he learns to fight
If he lives with fear, he learns to be anxious and insecure.

It he lives with pity, he learns to feel sorry for himself.

If he lives with ridicule, he learns to be shy.

If he lives with shame, he learns to feel guilty.

If he lives with encouragement, he learns to be confident in himself and his abilities.

If he lives with tolerance, he learns to be tolerant of others.

If he lives with praise, he learns to be appreciative.

If he lives with acceptance, he learns to love.

If he lives with approval, he learns to like himself.

If he lives with recognition, he learns that it is good to set goals for himself.

If he lives with security, he learns to have faith with himself and in other people.

<u>Key points</u>

- When organized comprehensive treatment strategies are planned great results can be expected.

- Parents should have an active role in the treatment strategy of their child.

- All treatments should be explored systematically and comprehensively.

- Medical help from qualified specialists and therapists should be sought.

- Parents should always be hopeful and optimistic.

20

BIOMEDICAL INTERVENTIONS

- What is the role of biomedical intervention in autism?

- What can be expected with biomedical interventions?

- Who is likely to respond to biomedical interventions?

- Are there any concerns about biomedical interventions?

- Are there useful guidelines when using a biomedical approach?

Biomedical intervention for our purposes is defined as treatments and therapies that involve use of biologically active agents either pharmacological or natural treatments that are thought to directly affect the body's biochemical system. For doctors who practice conventional medicine, drug therapy may be viewed as the only form of acceptable treatment. Alternatives therapies may be labeled as *unproven*. Although some pharmacological drugs do work, they may not be indicated to treat autism specifically. There is no FDA approved drug for autism as yet, though many drug companies are working hard to change that fact. The goal of this chapter is not to tell the reader which treatment option is best or most valid but simply to make the reader aware that there are various options that have been endorsed by qualified clinicians, and that many parents feel have played a significant role in the recovery of their child. Some of the more popular therapies are discussed in greater detail than others, but a full analysis of the different therapies is not my purpose in this chapter. If interested, further research can be done.

It is always important to do your own research. You should always, as a parent, seek to do what you think may be most useful for <u>your</u> child and do not be afraid to follow your instincts. Do not forget that an 'unproven therapy' may prove to be very useful for your child. Although there are false claims and a potential for financial exploitation, that should not deter parents from researching and trying different approaches. If anyone, even a physician, discourages you from looking for answers to viable treatment options, or maintaining hope, if that person cannot give you a safer and more effective therapy, do your own investigation.

PHARMACOLOGICAL INTERVENTION

Drugs may play a role in some cases. I personally do not believe that it is the best or safest option in most children with autism. Each case needs to be assessed individually. See the next chapter for a more detailed analysis on the role of drugs.

NUTRITIONAL INTERVENTION

Gluten-free casein-free (GF/CF) diet

Simply stated, this is a diet that is based on the notion that many individuals with autism are unable to tolerate wheat or dairy products. Therefore, these products are completely removed from the diet. Wheat products contain gluten and dairy derivatives contain casein. Both gluten and casein are proteins that many children with autism cannot digest properly. Instead of being broken down into the individual amino acid units needed for proper absorption, they are improperly processed. This leads to the formation of peptides (chains of amino acids, in particular gluteomorphins and casomorphins) that are neuroactive (can affect brain function, in adverse ways).

The affects include various behavioral, cognitive, and systemic problems. Common examples include frequent upper respiratory infections, ear infections, gastrointestinal complaints, inappropriate giggling, aggression, and hyperactivity, and a brain fog resembling a drunken state. This dietary intervention can work well if a child truly has a problem digesting gluten and casein appropriately, which is not the case for every autistic child. Children who have difficulties digesting these proteins may have disturbances such as zinc deficiency. Among other things, enzymes that digest these proteins (called peptidases) require zinc to do their job. In order for the GFCF diet to work well, the parents must be very strict with the diet. In some cases, even a minor infraction can prevent optimal benefits. The diet may take weeks (up to three weeks in the case of casein) or months (up to 3 months in the case of gluten) to work effectively. In individuals who do not seem to have a problem with casein, I still recommend avoiding dairy products because of the contaminants present such as hormones and antibiotics.

Specific Carbohydrate Diet (SCD)

This is a type of diet which removes starches and sugars (disaccharides and polysaccharides) from the diet allowing only honey and fruit sugars. The purpose is to eliminate the food source of harmful yeast and bacteria. The gut lining is expected to heal causing resolution of such symptoms as diarrhea or constipation. Initially developed for treatment of inflammatory bowel disease, many parents of children with autism have used the SCD.

DETOXIFICATION

A very important concept in biomedical intervention is that of detoxification. It is well recognized that many children with autism have problems with detoxification. Toxins vary in nature and include such things as heavy metals, yeast, environmental and food allergens, internal neurochemical substances from improperly degraded chemicals, or xenobiotics such as drugs. Detoxification is simply the process of removing unwanted chemicals or toxins from the body. Detoxification is an important process for everyone.

Chelation

Chelation is the removal of toxins, specifically heavy metals such as mercury. Chelation can be done pharmacologically using drugs (called chelators) that have the ability to bind and cause excretion of heavy metals from the body, or one can use natural means to encourage the bodies cells to detoxify on their own.

Chemical chelation

There are a variety of chelators used such as DMSA, EDTA and DMPS. The most promising chelation method to date in terms of safety and efficacy in dealing with mercury and arsenic in autism, according to some researchers, may be TD-DMPS or transdermal-dimercaptopropane 1-sulfonate. Many are using TD-DMPS in combination with glutathione, trandermally. Chemical chelation should always be done under the supervision of a qualified experienced physician such as a DAN! doctor.

Natural chelation

There are natural, non-pharmacological ways of encouraging the body to chelate itself. One of the best examples includes metallothionein promotion therapy. Researchers at the Pfeiffer Treatment Center in Illinois have found that many children with ASD have a dysfunctional protein called metallothionein. As indicated by its name, this protein is involved with metals. Specifically, it attracts metals like a magnet, ultimately resulting in their excretion. Dysfunction in this protein should be suspected in children who have high copper levels, low zinc, and a copper/zinc ratio greater than 1.2. This therapy consists in priming the body by providing it with extra zinc and other minerals and vitamins. Then the promotion of proper formation of the metallothionein protein is done by supplementing the body with 13 amino acids important in the synthesis of this protein.

BRAIN THERAPIES

Hyperbaric

Hyperbaric oxygen therapy (HBOT) is a way of administering pure oxygen in a pressurized chamber so that significantly more oxygen can be delivered to tissues than would normally be possible under normal atmospheric conditions. HBOT is thought to promote growth of new blood vessels, reduce swelling and inflammation, deactivate toxins, and speed the rate of healing. Initially used for decompression sickness, HBOT is being used to treat stroke, TBI (traumatic brain injury), CP (cerebral palsy), autism, MS, and CFS (chronic fatigue syndrome). There are 13 indications that are covered by federal programs for the use of HBOT, but there are a total of 66 applications for its use. Many individuals with strokes, cerebral palsy, and autism have used this form of therapy to try to reverse 'brain damage'. While several neurologists and clinicians endorse this form of therapy, it is still controversial. Many parents believe that it is an important therapy, the following parent who testified in front of the committee on Government Reform stated, "…the parent movement has taken on a life of its own. Desperate parents are going to continue to get HBOT for their children no matter what you decide today. Some are even talking about treating their children with scuba gear and 100% oxygen at the bottom of their swimming pools. We are crawling into chambers in the back of semis hidden on Indian reservations and in warehouses and having chambers installed in our homes. Parents are second mortgaging their homes and taking out huge unrepayable loans. Nothing can stop parents from getting HBOT for their children, but you can help us make it safe and available. We need studies to determine the safest and most efficacious protocol. The question is not whether hyperbaric oxygen therapy works. The exciting question is what other conditions will hyperbaric improve or cure" *2004 Hearing Autistic Spectrum Disorders: An Update of Federal Governmental Initiatives and Revolutionary New Treatment of Neurodevelopmental Disease.*

Vasodilation therapy

This is based on the notion that children with various neuropsychiatric conditions such as autism, Tourette's syndrome, ADHD, and learning disorders have symptoms that are caused by vascular blood flow problems. This therapy uses drugs that vasodilate blood vessels, thus increasing blood flow to the brain by reversing the constriction of brain vessels. This, therefore, should cause the symptoms to resolve. This therapy has traditionally been used for neurovascular conditions such as stroke, hypoxic injury, and other neurological conditions such as cerebral palsy. For further information visit the website: www.floridaneurologicalinstitute.com)

A word of caution to parents

Although I always advocate open-mindedness and a spirit of research, there are a lot of potential pitfalls when it comes to certain forms of treatment if one is not careful. Although I am very critical of organized medicine in certain respects, I am thankful for good science when it is upheld. There are therapies that are not yet well accepted because they are cutting edge and may later receive the proper attention from the scientific and medical community. There are, however, other types of treatments that are simply based on pseudoscience. There are therapies that survive remarkably well although they have little intrinsic value because they are fueled by the desperation of parents to try something new and because they may exert a placebo response (benefit from a therapy or agent with inert properties such as a sugar pill). See Chapter 26 for further discussion on this topic

Sample treatment approach that is safe and usually effective

Below I will outline a simple, organized approach that I consider reasonable. It is always important to work with an expert, although some basic things pertaining to general health can be initiated on your own. Some aspects of treatment can be generalized while others should be individualized based on clinical history and test results:

- First, correct nutritional problems. This means:

  - Eliminating foods that can lead to adverse affects:

    - Dairy products

      - In <u>some</u> cases one may need to be on a strict casein-free diet

    - Wheat may need to be removed in some patients

    - Caffeinated products

    - Red drinks

    - Excess refined sugar

    - Processed meats (especially red meats)

    - Foods that by experience or through food testing are shown to be a problem (either food sensitivities or allergies)

  - Supplement nutrients that may be deficient

    - Vitamins

    - Minerals

      - Especially zinc and magnesium

    - Antioxidants

    - Essential fatty acids

    - Amino Acids (if deficient based on testing)

    - Glyconutrients

    - Probiotics

    - Water (equivalent to half of the body's weight in pounds).

    - Fiber (obtained through fruits and vegetables)

- Correct the gut

  - Address problems with diarrhea or constipation.

  - Address possible yeast, parasites, or other microbial abnormalities.

  - Address the issue of increased gastrointestinal permeability.

  - Correct any reflux that may be present

- If a significant gastrointestinal problem is suspected, ask for a referral to the gastroenterologist.

- Strengthen the immune system

  - Antioxidants and other immune support agents may be necessary.

  - Remove toxins.

  - If a significant immune problem is suspected, ask for a referral to see an immunologist

- Look for and treat any seizure disorder present

  - See a neurologist (pediatric)

  - The neurologist should rule out other neurological problems

- Look for and treat any sensory processing disorder present

  - Central auditory processing disorder

  - Hyperacusis

  - Hearing impairment

  - Visual processing disturbances

  - Tactile defensiveness

  - Sensory integration dysfunction

- Appropriate referrals to specialists.

Parents and clinicians should remember that biomedical therapies usually fall under the rubric of either symptomatic treatment (where the goal is palliation) or restorative treatment (treating the underlying problem). In some cases a therapy may serve both purposes. The above statements apply for both pharmacological and non-pharmacological approaches. Drugs may be used to palliate symptoms or they may be used in an attempt treat the underlying problem (e.g. with chelation therapy or use of vasodilators).

The exact reason for a child's symptoms may not always be clear even if they respond to a given therapy that targets a particular response. Examples include chelation which includes heavy metal detoxification and concurrent supplementation of powerful antioxidants and useful minerals. Both of these may independently be useful in treating the child. Another example is with the GFCF diet. Patients that are placed on that diet, by the mere fact that they decide to go on such a strict diet, suggests that the parents are motivated to also improve the child's diet in general. Apart from the benefits of a casein-free diet, many may also be responding to the avoidance of dairy and its inherent contaminants. Many of the symptoms attributed to gluten and casein metabolites may also be due to other factors such as zinc deficiency, which itself can cause primary and secondary disturbances by itself.

Non-pharmacological therapies, I feel, are generally safer than drug treatment, especially for individuals with autism. This does not mean that these treatments are always safe or cannot cause problems. Experience with certain forms of chelation and the SCD for instance have been reported to show dramatic results in some children, but significant regression in others.

Key points

- There are a variety of biomedical options that can be used effectively to treat autism.

- Some biomedical interventions target symptoms and others target the underlying problem.

- Biomedical treatments used include both conventional and non-traditional approaches.

- Basic biomedical concepts that everyone can benefit from include proper nutrition, fixing the gut, strengthening the immune system and removing toxins.

- While some treatments involve general principles, others should be individualized for the particular child.

21

THE ROLE OF DRUGS IN AUTISM

- What types of drugs are used for autism?

- How safe are drugs for children with autism?

- If drugs are used, how long should they be used?

- What are the pros and cons of drug therapies for children with autism?

- What should be the role of drug therapy in autism?

Drug therapy is perhaps the most common conventional way medical doctors use to control autistic symptoms. Although at the time of the writing of this book, there are no FDA approved drugs for the treatment of autism, it is still a popular way of addressing autistic symptoms. There are specific reasons why patients with autism are treated with drugs. The most common reasons include:

- Behavioral problems
  - Aggressive behavior/excessive tantrums
- Neurological problems
  - Seizures
- Mental (psychiatric) conditions
  - ADHD
  - ODD (Oppositional Defiant Disorder)
  - Anxiety disturbances

- OCD

- General anxiety disorder

Examples of the common drugs and classes of drugs used include:

Antipsychotic agents (used for behavioral problems)
Antidepressants (used for OCD and anxiety disorders)
Selective Serotonin Reuptake Inhibitors (SSRIs)
Anticonvulsants
ADHD medications
Various other drugs are used based on symptoms present

Because drugs have to undergo a rigorous process before being approved and released, their mechanism of action, safety profile, and indication is *usually* well understood. For a subset of autism patients drugs do seem to work in palliating symptoms. The benefits of drugs in general include:

- They are well studied.

- They tend to have a quick onset of action (psychiatric drugs usually take longer to work).

- In many instances they may be covered by insurance companies.

- They are convenient.

- They are well accepted by the general medical community.

- They are undeniably the best option in acute situation (e.g. in acute situations such as a prolonged, life-threatening grand mal seizures or brain infection).

In the case of autism, drugs should be considered if:

- A potentially serious problem occurs like seizures that are epileptic in origin.

- Behavior that is out of control, especially if other treatments (.e.g. behavioral modification or nutritional therapies) have been tried unsuccessfully.

- Drug treatment for a particular problem is the safest, most effective therapy.

Unfortunately, there are limitations to drug therapy in autism and other neuropsychiatric conditions. These include:

• Drugs simply may not work for some individuals. Occasionally, drugs are tried (often concurrently) that cause a problem that was not there initially.

• Side effects may occur. Because children with autism often have sensitivities to a variety of substances (toxins, foods, common allergens), they are particularly vulnerable to medications. There is a subset of children with autism who are prone to develop tic disorders, and this may occur for the first time after they start taking a stimulant medication.

• Drugs do not address the underlying cause of autism even though they may help suppress the symptoms.

• Although some children appear to do well and tolerate certain drugs, the long-term consequences are not always clear.

• Indiscriminate use of drugs may cause a potentially correctable problem to be overlooked.

It is always best to search for the underlying cause(s) of a child's symptoms. Although drugs may help in selected cases, they should not be the first and only option given. The safest and most effective option should be used. Therapeutic approaches that are based on targeting the underlying defects instead of just suppressing the symptoms should be sought. When drugs are used, it is best if they are used for only a short time if possible. Monotherapy (use of only one drug) is safer than polypharmacy (use of multiple drugs concurrently). Additional drugs have sometimes been used to alleviate the side effects of another medication. Because some clinicians only focus on pharmacological interventions for autism, they end up using a drug for each symptom the child manifests. This can lead to the child being placed on a frightening number of medications. Drugs may be considered a treatment option for autism, but it is not the only option. It may be convenient, but they do not address the underlying issues in autism. Though effective, drugs may not always be safe.

Key Points:

• Drug therapy may have a role in the treatment of autism.

• When drug therapy is considered, it should be used wisely.

- Avoid polypharmacy and long-term medication use.

- Although there are benefits to drug therapy, there are limitations like side effects.

- Drug therapy even when used successfully, should not be a substitute for addressing the underlying condition.

- There are other options besides drugs.

22

REHABILITATIVE THERAPIES

- What is meant by rehabilitative therapies in autism?

- What is the rational for using rehabilitative therapies in biologically-based disorders?

- What types of therapies are available?

- How effective are rehabilitative therapies?

- How can rehabilitative therapies be made more effective?

I use the term *rehabilitative therapies* in connection with autism and other neuropsychiatric disorders to signify treatments that are based on repetition, reprogramming, or stimulation of brain pathways. In theory, these therapies work because of the principle of neuroplasticity. Brain connections can change with appropriate stimulation. Repetition, stimulation, and desensitization can affect the functioning of the brain. Many parents who have tried these therapies, report that they work.

Examples of rehabilitative therapies include:

    -Speech/language therapy (SLT)
    -Occupational therapy (OT)
    -Sensory integration therapy (SIT)
    -Auditory integration therapy (AIT)
    -Fast Forward
    -Tomatis
    -Sensory Learning

Some of these therapies last only for a few days (e.g. 10 days) and others are longer in duration. Occasionally the therapies will be repeated for better results. Apart from the primary benefits derived from these therapies, a secondary benefit includes the 'therapeutic touch'. In my experience, many therapists provide the type of kindness, care, and optimism that plays an important part in the success of a child with autism.

There are various other programs that are integrative and use approaches that help with brain development. One example is the National Association for Child Development (NACD). This is an eclectic program that is based on the philosophy that children with neurodevelopmental disorders can do well. This is based on a belief that these children have undeveloped potential. Parents are empowered to work with their children because they spend the most time with the child.

The more closely a therapy is directed to correlate with an autistic child's problems, the more likely it is that the child will have a good response to the treatment. For instance, a child with severe auditory processing problems may do well with a therapy that focuses on auditory processing abnormalities. If there is only partial improvement, then a child may have additional problems that have not been totally addressed by the therapy applied.

The specific type of therapy needed varies with each child. One child may do better with one type of rehabilitative therapy than another. Instead of looking for which therapy is 'the best' or 'most effective', it is more important to identify which therapy has the **best fit** for a particular child. I recommend that parents evaluate a given therapy carefully relative to the child's symptoms, and not based on reports of how another child has responded to the treatment since every child is different. Although some of the therapies listed above may be considered by some clinicians as 'unproven' in their efficacy, in my medical experience these therapies have been 'proven' to be effective for many patients and warrant further investigation. Many of the rehabilitative therapies help improve sensory processing function, which is an important component of the symptomatology in children with autism. Many secondary problems will resolve once the sensory processing problems are corrected.

Taking care of children with autism is like putting the pieces of a puzzle together. Each piece is important by itself, but also in so far as it fits into the larger picture. Some pieces must be laid down before the other pieces can be placed appropriately. Each piece is important, from the first to the last. The puzzle is not complete until each piece is in place. Initially, while the puzzle is being assembled, it may not make sense. As the picture nears completion, one can start to see what the whole picture looks like. Some puzzles are complex and take a larger amount of time. The more complex the puzzle, the greater the satisfaction when the puzzle is fully assembled. One should never be weary of putting the treatment pieces of autism together, for in doing so there are great rewards.

Key points

- Rehabilitative therapies focus on repetition, desensitization and reprogramming of brain connections, and should be considered in the treatment of autism.

- Rehabilitative therapies provide added benefit such as reinforcement of behavioral techniques.

- Rehabilitative therapies work because the brain is adaptable and subject to positive change.

- It is important to find which therapy is most suitable to your child.

- Treatment results vary depending on the child's needs.

- All interventions, rehabilitative therapies included, are pieces of a puzzle that must be assembled. In the case of autism, the final product is a restored child.

23

BEHAVIORAL INTERVENTIONS

- What types of behavioral interventions are available for children with autism?

- Can behavioral therapies correct a biologically disorder?

- How should children with autism be disciplined?

- What are the limitations of behavioral therapies?

- Is there a connection between behavioral and rehabilitative therapies?

Behavior problems are an important concern in individuals with autism. As mentioned earlier in Chapter 7, there are a variety of circumstances that can explain the behavioral problems seen in autistic children. These vary from cognitive, emotional, psychological, and psychiatric disturbances to biological derangements. The behaviors may sometimes be part of a coping mechanism, but not always. One question we would like to address in this section is how to differentiate between behaviors that are voluntary and involuntary In other words, how do we differentiate between 'WON'T' and 'CAN'T' in terms of behavior?

It is prudent to assume that a child 'CAN'T' control their behavior until proven otherwise. This means that behavioral problems should automatically trigger a search for a correctable underlying dysfunction. Always assume that a fit, tantrum, rage attack, or meltdown has a specific cause even if it apparently occurs 'out-of-the-blue' until you can prove that the behavior is within the child's control. Bare in mind that what may seem to be a trivial matter to you may have a strong impact on the autistic child.

Distinguishing between behavioral "WON'T" and "CAN'T"

"CAN'T" or involuntary behaviors:

- No obvious precipitant such as a child 'not having his way, following a change in routine, or another transition-related matter.

- Stereotyped behaviors or ones that are almost identical in nature and duration.

- Behaviors that occur at approximately the same time.

- Behaviors that only occur in a specific setting or during a specific activity.

- Behaviors that are preceded by, occur during, or are followed by a illness (for instance a streptococcal throat infection).

- Behaviors associated with an alteration consciousness.

- Behaviors associated with a specific gesture.

- Behaviors that do not respond to behavioral intervention or soothing mechanisms.

"WON'T" or non-compliant behaviors:

- Behaviors where an underlying problem has been ruled out.

- Behavioral outbursts with an identifiable trigger. The trigger may not be conspicuous. It may appear trivial.

- Behavioral problems that result from not getting what they want. The response may be prolonged and excessive, abnormally so. Maladaptive behaviors should be corrected as early and firmly as possible.

Children with autism apart from their disorder, have many areas in which they are like non-autistic children. Not every behavioral abnormality should be ascribed to psychopathology. Any two year old can have significant tantrums. Normal children can have some degree of defiance and oppositional behavior. Children have a normal range of personality traits that range from docile to rambunctious. Normal children can, for a variety of reasons, have fluctuations in their behavior. When these behaviors are excessive or abnormal, they require disciplinary measures. The following applies to these behaviors in children with autism and other disorders such as ADHD, oppositional defiant behavior, and related conditions.

The method used to discipline a child should be based on methods that allow a child to understand that the behavior is inappropriate and has adverse consequences. Because children with autism often have significant sensory processing limitations, it is important to utilize multi-sensory modalities in explaining and correcting behaviors. Providing verbal instructions only to a child who has severe auditory processing difficulties may be futile by itself. One may need to use visual cues, tactile demonstrations, and concrete examples. The concept is that one must be creative, and discipline children in a way that *they* can understand despite their sensory and cognitive limitations.

Consistency is always important in regards to disciplinary measures and is especially important for a child with autism. Children with autism are usually routine-oriented and do better with firm structure. Learning and behavioral management, therefore, require as much consistency as possible. Consistency should be present at home, school, and the homes of relatives. It is interesting to note that some children with behavioral problems only display these behaviors in settings where there is a lack of consistency and management of their behavior. In structured settings, they do not seem to manifest behavioral problems at all.

Disciplinary action must be delivered immediately! A behavior may more easily be extinguished if corrected right away. Again consistency is important when it comes to behavioral intervention. You will not get good results if you discipline intermittently. A disciplinary action should NEVER be delivered with anger, humiliation, or embarrassment for the child. This will only lead to further problems. Instead, firmness mixed with love, understanding, and a liberal amount of compassion should guide a parent's disciplinary actions. Some children with autism react differently to one parent than the other. It may appear that they can 'get away with more' with one parent. Usually that parent has a harder time providing effective discipline to the child. More firmness may need to be delivered by that parent to eliminate the discrepancy between the parents. Both parents should be viewed as authority figures and be able to correct the improper behaviors of the child. In situations where the behavior is unmanageable for the parents, it is appropriate to seek professional help. Any behavior that cannot be managed, even with the assistance of a behavioral expert, should prompt a search for an underlying medical problem.

Behavioral interventions are very popular, and are felt by many clinicians to play a crucial role in the treatment strategy of autistic children. Some clinicians even believe that these interventions are *the* most valuable therapies for children with autism. I believe that there is a strong role for behavioral interventions, but these should not be viewed as the only treatment strategy that is needed, or proven to work.

There are many behavioral intervention programs, but we will analyze one that has been well researched and is widely used. It is appropriately called Applied Behavioral Analysis (ABA). This is a therapeutic approach that ideally:

- Starts very early (before the age of four).

- Is very intensive (40 hours a week, 50 weeks per year, and for at least 2 years).

- Requires one-to-one behavioral treatment by a trained therapist.

- The treatment is geared toward improving behavior, language, speech, and social interaction skills.

The main approach in ABA is to breakdown various aspects of behavior into small, discrete, measurable units that are taught in small steps. Each step is taught by presenting an instruction. Prompts may be used to facilitate the process. Appropriate responses are followed by consequences that act as positive reinforcers. *Teaching trials* are used repetitiously, and their effects and progress recorded meticulously. The aim then of ABA is to help autistic children learn *how to learn* like normal children, and ultimately allow mainstreaming into regular school classes. The father of ABA is Ivar Lovaas. In order to understand this behavioral approach and its merits, let us look at Lovaas' origin and philosophy.

Dr. O. Ivar Lovaas was a professor of psychology at UCLA. He believed that autism was a psychological disorder, unresponsive to medical interventions. From his studies, he believed that autism could respond quite well to behavior modification interventions. Lovaas grew up in German occupied Norway, and wondered as a boy if the destructive actions of the Germans were genetic-based or environmental. This was the beginning of his interest in behavior that eventually led him to design his behavioral treatment of autism. He believed in the benefits of positive reinforcement. He presented the application of his theories back in the 1970s. He did long term studies in 19 young autistic individuals who received

4000 hours of intensive behavioral therapy. He started his research in 1963 when he examined, analyzed, and treated 20 children institutionalized at the UCLA Neuropsychiatric Institute. Interestingly, these children were between the ages of 5 and 12. Although these autistic children were severely affected, he found that with intensive behavioral treatment approaches, these children were actually able to learn abstract concepts. When these children left the institution, those who were placed in a non-conducive or unsupportive environment (like a state hospital), they lost all of the skills they had previously learned. However, those who went to more supportive and nourishing environments (their parents' home) maintained their skills. What Lovaas learned is that environment is extremely important, and can determine whether a child functions in a productive or destructive manner. He eventually moved from working in the 'controlled' hospital environment, to using a more natural setting like the homes of the children, where the parents could also be taught.

Lovaas/ABA, the good, the bad, and other lessons learned

Lovaas was very passionate and enthusiastic about his methods. Like other pioneers, he believed that his methods, if done early and intensively could reverse autism in many children. The questions that should be asked are the following: Was Lovaas' claims and studies accurate? Some have wondered if the initial 19 children that Lovaas studied were high functioning autistic children to begin with. Assuming that Lovaas' claims were accurate as well as the many studies that subsequently have replicated his findings, why do behavioral interventions have such a positive impact on a neurobiological disorder? The answer is addressed at the end of this chapter.

The most negative aspects of ABA have to do with factors that are now outdated. Lovaas admitted that in the 1960s, he used punishment or what was called 'contingent aversives' to control self-injurious behavior. The aversives included "smack on the butt" or "electric shock". These approaches were apparently successful, but tolerance soon developed requiring stronger aversives the next time. Although these techniques have rightfully been abandoned, Lovaas noted that many of these children engaged in very painful behaviors such as breaking their nose or poking their eyes. These same children, however, at the thought of an aversive would stop their self-injurious behavior, which is an interesting observation. The way an autistic child perceives things either good or bad will have a strong impact on their behavior.

Another limiting factor is the connection with operant conditioning. Basically this is a form of associative learning in which there is a contingency between the response and the presentation of the reinforcer. Operant conditioning has roots based on animal models, which I argue do not reflect the complexities of the human mind and human experience. ABA is related to the principles of operant conditioning, which has actually been used with some children with autism in the past. One critique is that the changes seen in autistic children treated with ABA, especially with respect to language, merely reflects parroting behavior. Others have argued that the rigorous long hours are not always necessary. Less stringent behavioral approaches may still yield good results.

In reality, behavior has an important vital role in autism. The main lesson to learn from ABA, and other forms of behavioral interventions, is that behavior is subject to change. Moreover, improvement of behavior is connected to learning and other cognitive aspects such as language. In a 1994 interview with Catherine Johnson as reported in the <u>Advocate</u>, Lovaas stated: "I don't claim a cure because we haven't gotten to the organic variable that is causing the autism. But the nervous system is pretty adaptable and with intensive therapy, the child may be able to work around his organic deviation". Behavioral interventions are based on the realization that change is possible. Neural circuitry and dendritic connections can change in the brain with insistent, persistent, and consistent treatments even if they are not biomedical. This is an encouraging property of the brain that it is subject to change. These treatments, however, should be employed in conjunction with biological approaches so synergistic improvement can be seen.

<u>Key points</u>

- Many children with autism have significant behavioral problems.

- It is always important to distinguish between won't (non-compliance) and can't (inability).

- Behavioral intervention therapies play an important role in the management of autism.

- ABA is an intensive form of behavioral therapy.

- The brain, and therefore behavior, is adaptive.

24

CLASSROOM THERAPIES

- What does classroom therapy entail?

- How does the educational experience affect children with autism?

- What educational programs are available for autism?

- What type of school is best suited for an autistic child?

- What should school teachers know about autism?

Educational strategies are an important component of autism treatment. Many young children with autism start to blossom socially after starting school. The right educational approach, however, is necessary. The reason why the educational system plays a vital role in autism is because children with autism can only learn when the environment is modified so that the child is able to comprehend and grow. This statement implies that children with autism do have the ability to learn given the right atmosphere.

Children with autism, as mentioned earlier, have a variety of sensory processing disturbances that affect the manner in which they learn. A child, who has significant auditory processing abnormalities, may rely on visual cues to assimilate information. The reverse might be true for an individual with significant visual perceptual limitations, but who has adequate auditory perceptual abilities. An educational program must recognize the particular academic needs of autistic children. A child who is able to learn and make sense of his or her environment is likely to improve not only cognitively, but also behaviorally and socially.

Another important aspect pertaining to education is the fact that children with autism require structure. Most autistic children are routine oriented. They get upset if there is an alteration in their routine. Why? Some children with autism are so sensory impaired (in terms of auditory perceptual, visual perception or both) that they require a consistent routine to make sense of their surroundings. They need to get their landmarks. If such a child is in a situation where the usual boundaries are missing, that child can get disoriented. This disorientation can lead to tantrums, self-stimulatory behaviors, or other problems. In a sense, structure and routine provide security for the autistic child. An educational program that recognizes these factors and provides the needed structure is one in which an autistic child can thrive. Children with other disorders such as ADHD or dyslexia may also do well with a structured routine-oriented approach to their education.

Children with autism have different strengths and gifts that are not usually recognized. Many children have an excellent memory, others have mechanically technical abilities, and yet others have amazing problem solving abilities. Some are artistic, while others show great aptitude for technological endeavors. If an autistic child's strengths are recognized and appropriately cultivated the child may improve in several respects. First, the child may be willing to open up and learn more if the area of their strength is explored. Self-esteem is another area that can be bolstered. This can promote emotional stability and growth. An area of strength can be used to compensate for weaker areas. Many children with autism have interests that are not always apparent. If their interests are not encouraged they may become frustrated, which can lead to behavioral problems. An educational program that capitalizes on a child's strength is likely to result in overall improvements.

There are many excellent educational models available. The purpose of this chapter is not to list and discuss each one but to demonstrate the usefulness of the educational approach. I will only mention two models: TEACCH and The Higashi School.

TEACCH (Treatment and Education of Autistic and related Communication handicapped Children) is a program based out of the University of North Carolina at Chapel Hill (in the school of medicine's psychiatry department). This was the first statewide, comprehensive, community-based program and was voted as "the most successful statewide program in the country" by the National Institute of Mental Health. The founder is Eric Schopler. TEACCH was developed in1974. The philosophy was to focus on the individual autistic child, his needs, interests, and skills. Structured teaching is viewed as the most essential mode of education. Independent work skills are emphasized as well as social and communication skills.

Another curriculum is the Boston Higashi School. This was developed by the late Dr. Kiyo Kitahara from Japan who developed the Daily Life Therapy. This program focuses on group dynamics and academic skills (mathematics and technology) designed for individual capabilities, art and music (to gain mastery and appreciation of aesthetics), and physical education (based on concepts of sensory integration and vestibular stimulation). The ultimate goal of the program is the development of self-care skills and eventually social independence.

The importance of these programs and similar ones is the realization of the uniqueness of children with autism, hence their special needs. By the same token, these children, in the right environment can learn when their strengths are recognized and utilized. It is also important to realize that learning is complex and dynamic. It involves sensory and cognitive processes that must function well for optimal academic and intellectual functioning. A program like Lindamood-Bell, which among other things highlights the role of mental imagery and verbal processing in comprehension, is a good example.

The question that usually arises when considering special educational programs for autism is whether these may not in fact deter a child from learning 'normal' behaviors. Some parents report that when their child was placed in an autistic school or a classroom with lower functioning children their child showed signs of regression and behavioral aggression. Which is better then, to mainstream autistic children or place them in specialized classrooms? The answer varies depending on the level of cognitive functioning of the child. The basic concept is for a given child to have his or her learning needs met in an environment which is conducive to learning and social development. Some higher functioning children may do well in a normal classroom setting with some modifications, such as the provision of an aide. The aide can be valuable in helping with the social interactions of the child. Many children with autism, even those that are higher functioning, may need prompting in social situations to improve their interactions with others and their environment.

Key points

- Educational interventions play an important role in autism and should begin early.

- Children with autism have the ability to learn in the proper setting.

- Many children with autism require consistent routine and structure.

- TEACCH is an example of a successful statewide educational program for autism.

- The choice of school for a child with autism should be individualized based on a child's particular needs.

25

FINDING APPROPRIATE SUPPORT

- When is support needed?

- What type of support is needed?

- What type of support is available?

- Where do you look?

- What are the different functions of a support system?

- What if no support is available?

Support is always needed when dealing with a child that has special needs, whether that child has autism, seizures, ADHD, or other neuropsychiatric condition. Support is usually available. One has to know where to look. There are various types of support that may be needed including moral support, medical support, financial support, and psychological support to name a few. Parents should never be scared to ask for support regardless of their station in life, level of education, or level of need. Let us look at some different types of support:

Psychosocial/moral support

This is perhaps the most important type of support needed. Having someone to provide moral support is invaluable. Support is important throughout the course of treatment. This support can come from family members. However, realize that relatives may not always be supportive for a variety of reasons. One reason is that they simply may not understand the nature or severity of the child's condition. Sometimes family members deny that there *is* a problem, or they may blame the parents for the child's problem. Sometimes people will blame 'bad parenting' for the child's condition. This is unfortunate since relatives should be there to build up the family and support the child. Relatives need to be educated about the child's condition.

An excellent source of support can be from the church or house of worship. A church that truly understands its mission should be an excellent vehicle to provide all types of support ranging from moral, financial, provision of respite care, etc. Friends, neighbors, and other acquaintances can also be a source of support. While they are providing support, this can be an excellent way for these individuals to learn more about autism. People that are involved in the care of a child with special needs have an excellent opportunity to learn about caring, patience, and sacrifice.

Local support groups are another excellent source of support. Autism support groups can be a forum for parents to share their experiences with others who are going through the same difficulties. The support groups are also a place where treatment information can be shared informally in an open, friendly environment.

Medical support

By medical support, I mean support in terms of medical information, assistance with treatment plans and strategies, proper evaluation, and anything pertaining to the diagnosis and proper management of ASD. I recommend the following medical support:

- Your primary care physician

- All medical specialists and therapists involved in the care of your child

- Early Intervention

- The Autism Society of America (ASA) [www.autism-society.org]

  - This site will give a lot of information on autism and statewide, federal and international resources

- Center For the Study of Autism [www.autism.com]

- Autism Research Institute [www.autismresearch.org]

  - In addition to research information, you can also obtain a list of DAN! practitioners

- Cure Autism Now (CAN) [canfoundation.org]

  - See resource page

There are many other excellent resources, but the above are a good place to start. The above websites each have multiple links. It is always important to be educated about autism as much as possible. As one branches out, one can find additional resources.

<u>Key points</u>

- Most families and parents of a child with ASD will need support.

- Never be embarrassed to ask for help.

- Seek support early.

- Support can be obtained from a variety of sources including friends, relatives, support groups and church.

- Psychosocial, moral as well as medical support is invaluable.

- There are various national organizations that provide useful resources.

26

TRADITIONAL AND ALTERNATIVE TREATMENT APPROACHES

- What is the traditional treatment approach for autism?

- Which treatment approaches can be considered alternative?

- Which type of approach is most effective?

- Can divergent approaches yield similar good results?

- Is it possible to bridge the gap between traditional and alternative treatment approaches?

Health care networks

I have had a unique experience in my medical training. While attending medical school I enrolled in a master's program in Health and Humanities and took a variety of courses in medical anthropology, medical geography, and medical sociology. My program allowed me to participate in projects that involved working with various clinicians from other medical fields such as naturopaths, chiropractors, aromatherapists, herbalists, and others. The opportunity to learn from these various health care practitioners *along side* the formal training I received in medical school was fascinating. While some clinicians have started out in one field, such as medicine and ended up going into another field such as naturopathy, I had the unusual opportunity to experience both concurrently in a critical stage of my education and training. I had ample opportunities to compare allopathic medicine with what is commonly referred to as alternative medicine. There are huge differences in the approach and philosophy used between allopathic and alternative medicine. There is often a strong antagonism between the different fields.

From my personal experience in working with different health care systems in the United States and abroad, I do not believe that any given system holds all the answers to treat all health-related conditions. Some systems have large ranges of available interventions and diagnostic capabilities, but there is a special niche for each reputable health care system. What this means for both clinicians and patients is that there should be a greater attitude of openness and acceptance. Clinicians should employ a referral system between the different health care systems. There should be open and free communication between the different medical practitioners. Instead, each health care system believes they are prepared to deal with all medical problems, and considers the other systems to be inferior. Things are changing, but very slowly. Complex conditions such as autism require an interdisciplinary approach between various health care systems.

Very few medical conditions fuel the type of controversies as encountered with autism. The controversies raise serious questions. Well trained physicians and researchers fall on both sides of the fence. The families of children with autism are caught in the middle of the conflict. They are already overwhelmed, and are simply looking for safe effective treatment options for their children. Controversies can serve a useful purpose, however, in that they allow us to consider both sides of an issue and to understand the subtleties of the controversy that would otherwise remain hidden.

With respect to the types of treatments, some are conventional and others are considered alternative. It may not be easy to define what a conventional treatment for autism is since the very nature and cause of autism is heavily disputed. Therefore, different approaches are used in its treatment. Because neuroscientists believe that autism is caused by a defect of the developing brain resulting in life long deficits, treatment, based on this understanding would be palliative primarily. Indeed, organized medicine deals with autism by addressing its symptoms. The easiest way for this to be done is by using drugs. Drugs are used because of the studies and scientific research conducted. They can be prescribed only by physicians. Drugs therefore, can be considered the most conventional of medical treatments for autism, at least by physicians. Apart from drugs, behavior modification therapies and educational approaches have gained a level of acceptance that may place them in the same category of general acceptance as drugs. Speech and language therapy can be considered conventional treatments. Everything else is generally viewed as being non-conventional.

Non-traditional therapies and treatment modalities should not be regarded as inferior or ineffective. They are simply ones that have not yet gained full acceptance by the scientific medical community at large. What is now considered *snake oil* may eventually be accepted as standard therapy. What is presently regarded as standard accepted medical treatment *now* may later be regarded as a flawed improper therapeutic approach. Unfortunately, there are clinicians and researchers who have discovered useful interventions that are presently considered to be on the fringes of medical therapy. These individuals may in fact be ahead of their time. Their work, though, may not be validated for years to come.

The problem is that pseudoscientific therapies are placed in the same category as non-traditional therapies. These therapies have the appearance of being scientific and gain some degree of credibility, but then there is no scientific substance to their theories. These pseudoscientific therapies still thrive because they are aided by a placebo response. A placebo is an inert substance that when taken has a therapeutic effect. These therapies can be made to appear as authentic as other accepted therapies. There is a fine line between promising bona fide treatments and those that are invalid pseudoscientific and based on fraud. Both may be considered 'unproven' as far as the general medical community is concerned, but only one may possibly hold the key to the future treatment of autism.

Consider alternative therapies if conventional ones are not helping or if the alternative therapies are safer. Because of the potential for misleading therapies, one should proceed with caution. Pseudoscientific, fraudulent therapies are ones that may be:

- Very expensive

- Theories based on a flawed understanding of science

- Work for every known disorder, i.e. cure-alls.

- Require little or no formal training to administer.

Traditional versus non-traditional treatment approaches in autism is partly based on the different ways people understand the disorder. Autism is embedded with controversies, which lead to the establishment of different opposing paradigms. We will consider these controversies.

Controversies in autism

- The importance of environmental factors versus genetic predisposition

- The actual incidence and prevalence of autism

- Autism as an epidemic

- The role and safety of vaccines in autism

  - Thimerosal (mercury) and autism

  - MMR vaccine in autism

  - Other environmental, iatrogenic factors

- The role of nutritional and other biomedical interventions

- The reversibility of autism

Statistics on autism:

- Prior to 1980 the incidence of autism was believed to be approximately 4-5 per 10,000 for broader autistic spectrum disorders (1/10,000 for classic ASD). The incidence of autism may now be as high as 6/1000 (or 1/150) in some areas.

  - (CDC, April 2000 "Prevalence of Autism in Brick Township, New Jersey, 1988: Community report"; Report on Autism to the California Legislature)

- There was a 210% increase in the diagnosis of autism in California children over an 11-year period.

  - (*US. News & World Report,* June 19, 2000, p.47).

Based on these alarming statistics the following conclusions have been reached:

- More recent studies found that the rate of autism was higher than the rates from studies conducted in the United States during the 1980s and early 1990s. JAMA 1-Jan-2003; 289(1):49-55 (A study looking at the prevalence of autism in a major US metropolitan area-Atlanta).

- Based on reviews of the available literature surveyed, there is evidence of large increases in the prevalence of autism in both the US and the United Kingdom "that cannot be explained by changes in diagnostic criteria or improvements in case ascertainment". Blaxil MF—Public Health Rep-01-NOV-2004; 119 (6): 536-51.

- "In recent years concern has been shown about the possible increase in the prevalence of ASD. Studies have shown an increase, but during these last 20 years, diagnostic criteria and definition have also changed. Although many factors are at play, it is evident that there has been an increase". Merrick J—Int J Adoles Med Health—01—Jan—2004; 16 (1):75-8

- According to one study, autism is more common in males, multiple births, blacks, increased maternal age and increased maternal education. J Autism and Developmental Disorders 01—June-2002; 32 (3):217-24

All of the above studies suggest that autism is on the rise. Other studies, however, have suggested that there is no major change in the incidence of autism if you correct for certain factors:

- The rates in recent surveys are substantially higher than 30 years ago merely reflecting the adoption of a much broader concept of autism, a recognition of autism among normally intelligent subjects, changes in diagnostic criteria, and an improved identification of persons with autism attributable to better services. Pediatrics Vol. 107 No. 2 February 2001, pp. 411-412.

- "There is evidence that changes in case definition and improved awareness [of autism] explain much of the upward trend of rates in recent decades". Fombonne E—J Autism Dev Disord-01-AUG-2003; 33(4):365-82.

The principle issue of contention in the debate over the increased incidence of autism has to do with possible underlying etiologies. If the incidence of autism is truly increasing at the alarming rate suggested, it means the following:

-Whatever role genetic factors play in the etiology of autism, environmental triggers play an even bigger role.
-If environmental factors play a role, one has to look for environmental changes that have occurred in the past 2 decades, since that is when the sharp rise in the incidence of autism has been noted.

The most obvious changes in the past couple of decades have included:

- Increased environmental pollution and toxic exposures.

- Increased usage of Thimerosal (a preservative is some vaccines that contains ethylmercury) as the number of required vaccines for children has increased.

If the above is true, then clinicians, researchers and politicians must work together to investigate the problem, which may in part be iatrogenic and correct it immediately. If, on the other hand, the argument that suggests that there is no real increase in the incidence of autism is true, the following applies:

- There is no need to alarm people about the aforementioned environmental factors in connection with autism.

- Any treatment protocol, based on correcting purported environmental triggers must be erroneous, such as chelation (removing mercury from the body originating from Thimerosal).

- Although more research on autism is needed to determine the cause, the main focus should be on genetics, even if environmental factors play a minor role.

As we mentioned earlier, parents are caught in the middle of the controversies. In a practical sense, parents of children with autism want to know if it is safe to vaccinate their children. What are the risks? What should be done if a vaccine (Thimerosal) injury is suspected? These concerns are valid. Are vaccines safe? Have they contributed to a rise in the incidence of autism? Some studies have suggested that there is no significant link between autism and Thimerosal. Most pediatricians at this time do not believe that vaccines play any significant role in the etiology of autism. Some pediatricians are angered by these discussions because they feel that this sort of controversy will lower compliance rates for vaccination with grave infectious disease consequences to our communities. Let us look at both sides of the argument concisely and offer recommendations.

Arguments suggesting vaccines/Thimerosal is safe and unrelated to autism:

-Most children who are vaccinated do well and do not develop autism.
-There is no scientific proof that the cumulative amount of ethylmercury in Thimerosal contained vaccines cause brain injury resulting in autism.

-Genetic studies are increasingly revealing the important role of genetics in autism

> HOXA1 gene and autism
> 7q22-q33 and autism
> 15q11-q13 and autism

Arguments suggesting vaccines/Thimerosal may be related to autism:

-A study by Dr. Amy Holmes looking at mercury levels in first baby hairs revealed that the levels of mercury were significantly <u>lower</u> in children with autism, suggesting a mercury detoxification impairment. This in turn was felt to result in higher intracellular accumulation of mercury and organ and brain dysfunction.

-A study entitled <u>Neurotoxic effects of postnatal Thimerosal are mouse strain dependent</u> revealed that autoimmune disease sensitive mice subjected to Thimerosal challenges similar to that in the routine childhood immunization schedule, showed various neurological and neuropathological changes that were not present in other strains of mice without the autoimmune sensitivity. This study suggested that individuals with an autoimmune genetic diatheses may be at risk for the development of autism when exposed to Thimerosal.

-It has been noted that a significant subset of individuals with autism have family members with autoimmune disorders.

-The Journal of Pediatrics in November of 2002 published a study entitled <u>Increased prevalence of familial autoimmunity in probands with PDD.</u> The conclusion in that study was that: "Autoimmunity was increased significantly in families with PDD compared with those of healthy and autoimmune control subjects (*those without PDD*). These preliminary findings warrant additional investigation into immune and autoimmune mechanisms in autism".

-In the past, some children exposed to mercury via teething lotions and other mercury containing compounds developed "Pink's disease". These children with Pink's disease had some characteristics similar to autism, including sensory hypersensitivities, various neurobehavioral problem, and acrocyanosis. With the removal of mercury, the occurrence of Pink's disease declined. This suggests that mercury in young infants can lead to autistic-like symptomatology. Some children were noted to be particularly sensitive to the mercury, and others not all.

Given the above information, it seems clear that:

-Autism has a genetic component.
-Many children with autism have an autoimmune genetic diathesis.
-Some children with autism may have a particular genetic pre-disposition placing them at risk for Thimerosal/mercury toxicity.

A parent of a child with autism who has a family history of autoimmune diseases should be cautious and discuss the above concerns with their physician.

Are controversies bad? I believe that controversies are useful because they allow us to consider different aspects of an issue. Usually there are elements of truth on both sides of the discussion. The problem is that these elements are used and interpreted in a framework or paradigm that the opposite side might disagree with. Although truth is absolute, our understanding and interpretation of truth may be relative, and may sometimes be corrupted by personal worldviews or hidden political agendas.

In the case of autism, I believe that there *is* better awareness of the disorder. Many movies and books on autism (e.g. Rain-man) have popularized a disorder, which a few decades ago was not well known. There have also been changes in the criteria that allow more individuals to be classified as autistic. Many children with autism today do not fit Kanner's criteria for autism. They may show more affection and not demonstrate problems from birth. Despite the above, I still believe that autism is on the rise independent of the change in diagnostic criteria and better awareness of the disorder. That environmental factors play an important role is indubitable. Genes themselves can be affected by environmental factors. What that means is that beyond understanding the role of genes, which is important, researchers should focus more on the various environmental triggers present and see how they may alter gene function. Researchers should also try to understand how particular genetic alterations, mutations, and dysregulation problems translate into clinical symptoms. This line of study, I believe, would be more useful than trying to find a better, less toxic drugs to treat autism and its related disorders.

For now, it may be wise to:

- Postpone all vaccinations when the child is ill.

- Spread out the vaccine schedule (avoid taking too many vaccines at once).

- Supplement the child's diet with multivitamins and antioxidants prior to the vaccination for extra protection.

- Use Thimerosal-free vaccines (always check).

- Any neurological, immunologic or systemic changes noted after the vaccines should be reported right away. If a connection is suspected, treatment should be started right away (see Chapter 20).

See Appendix C for further recommendations on vaccines.

PARENTS AND PHYSICIANS

PARENTS AND PHYSICIANS SHOULD WORK TOGETHER TO HELP SOLVE THE AUTISM CRISIS! Physicians should be better listeners when it comes to autism. They should be good educators and teachers. In fact, the Latin word for doctor, *doceo* is *to teach.* They should be more aware of the role of nutritional therapies in autism, and other disorders in general. They should be more open-minded to theories and ideas that were not taught in medical school, if they are plausible. Parents should not look down on physicians simply because they are not as well informed about particular treatment options. It is true that many physicians are close-minded when it comes to autism treatments of which they have never heard. New ideas that go against what physicians have been taught are very hard for doctors to accept or even consider, especially if they are not validated by well-designed, double-blind, placebo-control studies.

When it comes to obtaining help from your doctor for your child with autism, keep the following in mind:

- Be assertive but not aggressive.

- Do not be defensive or antagonistic.

- Be persistent but not overly demanding.

- Propose but do not impose.

- Ask questions.

- If you would like your physician to consider a particular treatment approach, find studies to support the effectiveness the treatment to give to your physician.

- It is appropriate to request a referral to a specialist, or ask for a second opinion if you do not feel that your physician is addressing your concerns.

- It is always better to work with a physician that may not be as knowledge about autism but is open-minded and willing to help than one that says they know a lot but are close-minded about alternative treatment options.

Be cognizant that controversies exist. When medical controversies cannot be resolved easily, it may mean that there are some truths on both sides. There may be political issues involved, and confusing data that make the information subject to multiple explanations. You must do what you feel is best for your child bearing in mind safety concerns. Traditional medicine, unfortunately, is not always as open as it should be to nutritional non-pharmacologic biomedical interventions. However, with non-conventional therapies the door is sometimes left open so wide that there is room for a lot of charlatans, greedy opportunists, and pseudo-scientists to creep in, preying on helpless patients, their desperate parents, to obtain their money. Parents should therefore always be on the alert.

Before starting a particular treatment/therapy, ask the following questions:

1. How long will the treatment/therapy last?

2. What is the anticipated outcome?

3. What are the best and worst case scenarios?

4. What are the possible side effects?

5. How long should a particular treatment be continued, before deciding that it is not helpful for the child?

6. Why was that particular treatment chosen for your child?

The ideal treatment is one that is effective, safe, affordable, reasonable and doable.

<u>Key points</u>

- There are a variety of traditional and non-traditional therapies used in autism.

- Both traditional and non-traditional therapies may be effective or futile depending on the situation.

- Non-traditional interventions may sometimes include therapies that utilize pseudoscientific principles. It is important to investigate all claims made.

- Many controversies exist regarding treatment options, there may be elements of truth on both sides.

- It is advisable to be open-minded, but cautious when it comes to treatment options.

27

THE MISSING LINK AND THE RESTORATION MODEL

- What are the most important questions when it comes to autism?

- Is autism curable?

- Can restoration occur?

- Are there deeper issues that should be explored beyond biological one?

- Is there a role for spirituality in the understanding and management of autism?

THE RESOTORATION MODEL

Meaning of Restoration

The Restoration Model is based on the concept that a return to normal health is possible. There must be some deviation from normal in order for illness to occur. In the case of neurodevelopmental disorders, the deviation can occur before birth, during the perinatal period, or during the first few years of life. The deviation from normal can be caused by many factors. These factors affect the victim through some form of trauma, which results in either dysfunction or damage. Although the initial impact of the trauma can result in dysfunction, reparation, healing, and prevention of secondary problems is possible. It is always important, however, to identify and treat the effects of the primary problem in order for restoration to occur. Traumatizing insults can be physical, emotional, psychogenic, spiritual, or a combination of these. Restoration necessitates fully addressing each area involved from the trauma. The Restoration model is based on the simple assumption that the body, including the brain, has the intrinsic ability to heal itself. A person can return to normal (health) if the underlying problem(s) and

151

their secondary affects are corrected. In order to affect this healing, though, we must use the proper effective tools/equipment. Think of a skilled surgeon who has a faulty scalpel; he may not be able to carry out his task well despite his skills as a surgeon if his scalpel is dull.

The Restoration model would be incomplete and limited if it did not also include one very important external consideration. Although restoration can occur in many cases, including ones that have been labeled as refractory, based on the above principle, something may still be lacking. The missing factor is the dependency on Divine intervention. According to the Restoration model, there may be situations where restoration is only possible through direct intervention from God.

Quick fix

Quick fix solutions in autism and other disorders would be possible only if, one were to identify the particular trigger or set of triggers and correct them immediately using the most appropriate interventions. The problem is that this usually does not happen. In the case of autism, for example, even when a child is taken expediently to their physician, sometimes there are delays due to uncertainty regarding the nature of the problem. Even when a problem is quickly identified, however, the outward symptoms may have been developing subclinically (silently) for a significant amount of time. In the case of infections, we call this the *incubation period*. If one is exposed to a virus for instance, that virus may start to replicate and elicit an immune response several days or weeks before symptoms are noticed. If detected very early one may abort the infection before it ever becomes a problem. In the case of autism and other neuropsychiatric disorders, not only is the initial insult not picked up early in most cases, but various secondary problems develop before the diagnosis is made making the initial insult somewhat elusive to treatment. By the time the symptoms are finally recognized and therapy is begun, one has to correct various secondary disturbances that have developed in addition to the initial problem. Therefore, a quick fix should not be the goal of treatment as it is often not possible. Although a quick fix may not be possible in most cases of autism, full restoration should be sought even though time and effort may be required. The course is generally longer, the older the child is when treatment is finally begun. Despite the age of the child, one should never give up hope. Some of my oldest patients were started on therapies when they were over 30 years old, and are progressing well.

The Time element

Many children with autism who are on the right track as far as treatment is concerned may only require more time for recovery to occur. The concept of patience has become all too foreign to us today. Restoration is possible when the right elements are present, but it takes time. The progression may be slow, but the child should be noted to be improving. If there is no progress being made, then the treatment strategy needs to be re-evaluated. The element of time, may be a significant missing link in some situations. Parents must give each therapy an appropriate amount of time to be effective. Often parents will become anxious, and will switch between different therapies without given any of them time to work successfully upon the child.

Therapeutic mergers and new solutions

There are many reports of individuals with autism who with early, aggressive, and appropriate treatment have improved so much that they no longer meet the criteria for the diagnosis of autism. The therapeutic interventions that affect these improvements are from varied fields such as behavioral, educational and biomedical. This suggests that different modalities can provide beneficial results that may be helpful although divergent in nature. In many other cases, however, there are children with autism who have tried many different therapies, spent time, resources, and energy but to no avail. These 'refractory' cases require a search for a missing link. A child with autism who has persistent symptoms despite the implementation of various therapies has either not found the right therapy, or has a <u>seemingly</u> irreversible problem. I use the term "seemingly" because, as we shall see, 'irreversible', 'refractory', 'intractable' and 'incurable' are all relative self-imposed terms.

First let me summarize the information that we have on the causes of autism and its clinical findings:

1. Autism has a genetic component. There is not just one but several genes that are involved with autism.

2. Genetics alone do not explain the full clinical picture. Non-genetic environmental causes play an important role.

3. Autism is a neurodevelopmental and neurobiological disorder which usually begins before the age of 3. The developing brain at that time is vulnerable to certain insults that cause dysregulation of neurons that subsequently affects the brain in specific areas.

4. Neuropathologic and radiographic studies show evidence that the brain is affected in several areas, mainly the temporal and frontal lobes.

5. Immune mechanisms are demonstrated in many cases of autism, and inflammatory changes in neurons and neuroglia (supporting cells) have been noted.

6. Children with autism have significant language, behavioral, and social issues which interfere with normal functioning. They have the ability to learn and improve despite the presence of brain dysfunction. This suggests that despite the presence of subtle brain abnormalities in children with autism; these may be one of <u>many</u> risk factors and dysfunctions that contribute to the picture of autism. The relative contribution of these lesions may vary from one individual to the next.

With respect to treatment, IT IS A MISTAKE TO ASSUME THAT ONE PARTICULAR APPROACH, WHETHER BIOMEDICAL, BEHAVIORAL, EDUCATIONAL, ALTERNATIVE THERAPY IS <u>THE</u> ONLY APPROACH THAT IS EFFECTIVE OR THAT SHOULD BE CONSIDERED FOR A CHILD. When a child does remarkably well with one system, it is because that particular child might have a problem that responds best to that specific treatment modality. One treatment modality may also enhance another area of intervention. Imagine a severely affected child with autism, whose seizures, malnutrition and metabolic defects are corrected. That child may not only show significant overall improvement, but specific changes in learning, other cognitive functions and behavior should be expected. Any other therapies the child is receiving would be expected to work better and faster.

So what is the missing link? Every child may have a different missing link or set of missing links. I believe that more children with autism would recover if the right approach for that child were chosen. The belief that autism is incurable is one that is based on an underestimation of the intrinsic ability of the body and brain to heal itself. There are of course factors that have to be taken into consideration such as:

- Getting an early diagnosis.

- Starting treatment as soon as possible.

- Finding the right treatment.

- Being compliant with a given treatment.

- Using a multi-model system of treatment.

- Being open-minded, patient and optimistic.

One area of concern mentioned earlier, is the fact that since autism is such a complex disorder with still a lot of unknowns, this encourages the development of scam, pseudoscientific and exploitative treatments. Despite the above fact, one still has to remain open-minded. Some pseudoscientific therapies, if given with love, enthusiasm and delivered in a manner that fosters optimism, may actually be more effective than a conventional and 'proven' therapy that is delivered in a cold pessimistic manner. Even pseudoscientific therapies sometimes may have an important wedge of truth even if that truth is overblown and exaggerated. The famous French author Voltaire, once observed: "*Il semble que toute superstition ait une chose naturelle pour prinicipe, et que bien des erreures soient nees d'une verite dont on abuse*". The translation is: "It seems that behind all superstition, there is a natural principle but errors are borne out of a truth that is abused".

I worry about scientific inquiries that ignore a line of research simply because it is novel. In the case of autism we must try to investigate everything we can about the disorder but from different aspects. There needs to be collaborative efforts at research from various health care systems. It is interesting to note that in certain leading academic institutions such as MIT, researchers in computer science and technology were amazed to find out what happened by combining two very different fields of endeavor. Although each field had solved bits and pieces of a complex problem, by combining the two fields, new answers were formed and with much greater accuracy. The same applies with autism. Different medical paradigms must breakdown their barriers and communicate with each so that new more effective solutions can be found.

It is encouraging to note that autism has become such an important problem and has received so much attention, that a lot more research is now underway. Collaborative efforts are made with several leading academic institutions. I believe that by being objective and open-minded, these researchers can start to investigate some theories that right now are considered to be on the edge. In some cases, I predict that research will show that several of these therapies are indeed beneficial. It will be amazing to see what happens when an official seal of approval is given to some interventions that were previously discarded by the conventional medical establishment. I believe this will happen.

Perhaps the main concern though for parents of children with autism is simply finding out what can be done to help their child now! While theories are important and understanding the underlying pathophysiology of the disorder is interesting, parents are concerned with discovering what the best treatment options are for their child. They would prefer to find a systematic, sensible, and safe treatment plan that is not financially prohibitive. Dubious authority figures, such as 'Dr. Internet', can be informative, confusing, overwhelming, and misleading. For those families who are 'at the end of their rope', what can be done to help their children recover? Is there reason to hope for a recovery? Is such a thing possible? That is what we want to address in this last section of the book, which I consider the most important.

The Restoration model

I have developed a model called the **RESTORATION** model. The term "RESTORATION" was chosen since it describes the intent of the model, which is total re-establishment of health and wellness. I use this model not only for autism, but also for other complex neurological and neurobehavioral conditions. I wish to show below how total restoration is possible.

This model is based on the following premises:

- Humans are created beings. God is the Creator and is all powerful, all loving and all knowing. He is the ultimate healer.

- God has created each one of us with self-healing bodies. We are fully equipped with all the tools, processes, and the wisdom necessary to heal ourselves when we are sick.

- We are complex beings with a body, mind, and soul. We have emotional and spiritual needs as well as more tangible bodily requirements. A disturbance in any of these areas can affect all the others.

- God has given us a set of natural laws, regulations, and guidelines that promote wellness. This is a specific owner's manual to total wellness.

- Violation of these natural, God-given health laws place us at great risk for all types of malfunction (spiritual, physical, behavioral, psychiatric or emotional).

- We are designed to be healthy and live long, happy productive lives. Disease and illness are never haphazard, accidental events.

- Total restoration is always possible. Although in some cases it would take a miracle. God may in some situations allow illness to occur for the greater good of a patient or family. God is never the author of pain or sickness. He may allow illness to occur temporarily.

- Submitting entirely to God's will and His laws is the best way to ensure total restoration. This submission, itself, can be therapeutic. We need to rely upon His will.

- Because total restoration is possible, one should always maintain an optimistic and hopeful attitude. Patience is required.

Traditional or conventional approaches are limited when it comes to complex conditions like autism. Focusing primarily on biological disturbances, genetic factors, neurological impairments, or other biomedical malfunctions is restrictive. Countless parents of children with autism have been told that the only reliable and proven treatment options are drugs, along with proper educational placement. No real hope of a cure is provided to the parents. Instead, they are told that the child will probably never improve enough to lead an independent productive life. Some parents are told to institutionalize their child. This has in fact been a common practice in the past. Many parents are warned to stay away from any treatment option that includes nutritional interventions because they are not proven to work. Parents are told what approaches to avoid, but not what to *do* to overcome autism. Autism is not viewed as a curable condition. Officially, autism is viewed as a developmental disorder with an unknown etiology, and no known treatment options beyond simple palliation.

The conventional model of medicine as used in general practice today is great in many respects but faulty in others. The medical system in this country is considered by most to be the best in the world, but it is has limitations. This is apparent in conditions like autism, which is commonly viewed as being incurable. Most children with autism have normal brains structurally, at least based on tests like *routine* MRIs. Some cases may appear refractory because they are viewed from a limited biologically-based paradigm, the present conventional biomedical model. Understanding biomedical factors are vital. In my opinion, these biomedical factors should be understood in the context of normal body physiological function. There is an over-reliance on pharmacological intervention. Ignoring the body's ability to overcome its limitations when it comes to autism, points to ignorance of the amazing abilities of the human faculties.

In the **RESTORATION** model, we expand the biomedical framework into a biopsychosociospiritual construct. In this construct, biological derangements, which can be congenital or acquired, can alter mental function. But the reverse is *also* true. Acquired or secondary mental disturbances can alter biological function. The immune system is altered by and consequently impacts both biological and mental function. Mental disturbances can impair immune function also. Social factors, though external, can also affect health, through their effects on the individual's emotional well-being. Most important, and unique to the **RESTORATION** model, is the central role of *spiritual* factors. The ultimate determination of health and wellness is God's healing power. The spiritual component introduces such concepts as faith, prayer, and divine submission. It is the spiritual component of this model that makes total restoration possible even in cases that are labeled as *incurable, intractable, or refractory*. Because this model is based on the premise of a living, all-loving, and all-powerful Creator, true hope is always encouraged.

Now let us look at the individual components of the **RESTORATION** model more closely.

The doctor within and the RESTORATION model

Albert Schweitzer, noted author, physician, missionary and Nobel laureate, once wrote: "It's supposed to be a secret, but I'll tell you anyway. We doctors do nothing; we simply encourage and help the doctor within". When an ailment is present, one should look for the underlying cause and focus on *it* for proper treatment. It does not make much sense to treat a condition or symptom, simply by masking its expression. For example, if someone has headaches that are severe and recurrent, there are two options. One is to take ibuprofen each time the headache occurs. In this first option, one might even take a preventive daily pill to treat the headaches. By either taking an abortive pill or a preventative medication, the drug taken is just treating the pain, not the underlying problem causing the pain. Ibuprofen makes your headache go away, but this does not mean that your headache was caused by an ibuprofen deficiency. The ibuprofen simply blocked a pain pathway, thereby causing relief to occur. It is important to mention, however, that taking ibuprofen regularly can lead to rebound headaches where the medication itself causes 'analgesic rebound' headaches.

An alternative approach to treating the recurrent headache disorder is to seek the underlying cause for the headaches and treat it directly. The cause may be related to nutrition, like the consumption of migraine food triggers (caffeinated products or processed meats containing nitrates). Another cause may be nutritional deficiencies such as magnesium or riboflavin. And lastly, the cause may be from a particular food allergy. Headaches can be due to poor lifestyle choices, sleep deprivation, or stress. Addressing these underlying problems can cause the headaches to go away safely. This does not mean that drugs cannot be used, but this option should be used temporarily and viewed as palliative instead of curative. Identifying the underlying problem and treating it appropriately *can* lead to a cure.

Another example is someone who is always sick with recurrent pharyngitis and upper respiratory infections. One option is to repeatedly prescribe antibiotics, which leads to further problems. Conversely, one can focus on boosting the immune system by avoiding foods that are allergenic and overly processed, while increasing the intake of foods rich in vitamins, minerals and antioxidants. The latter is natural and safer.

Take the example of a sickly child with multiple allergies, behavior problems, seizures, headaches, and insomnia. One option is to place the child on multiple drugs. One drug for behavior and a second to counter the specific side effects of the first drug, a third drug to help the child's sleep disturbance, a fourth one for seizures, a fifth drug for the headaches and a sixth drug for treatment of allergy symptoms. A seventh drug is later added to counter the side effects caused by the various drug-drug interactions. This example may seem extreme, but polypharmacy is fairly common. A better option is to use *the doctor within* to take care of all of the child's problems, which may be interrelated. The child may have headaches and seizures that disturb his behavior and sleep, and because of their severity he develops a secondary mood disorder. Using proper nutrition, dietary supplements, avoidance of junk food, and awareness of psychosocial stressors that can contribute to sleep disturbances, headaches and mood disturbances it is possible to control the child's problems.

The popular conventional medical approach of relying on pharmacological intervention as the ultimate solution for everything is unwise. There is virtually a drug for everything. If you are overweight, there is a drug. If you are underweight, there is another drug. If you are sad, there is a drug. If you are mad, another drug exists. If you cannot fall asleep or if you sleep too much, there are drugs for that also. However, all drugs have side effects, sometimes they are identical to the conditions that they are designed to treat. Drug therapy can be considered as the *band-aid approach.* When you are bleeding, a band-aid is applied *temporarily* to allow the body to heal itself by allowing the blood to clot. Once this occurs, the band-aid can be removed. The band-aid did not actually do any healing itself. It stopped the bleeding mechanically temporarily, while allowing the body's coagulation cascade to perform its job. Drugs, like band aids, may serve a temporary purpose, but the healing ultimately must come from within the body.

Children, for instance, who are hyperactive, oppositional, and aggressive, may be started on stimulant medications without having their actual underlying problem fully addressed. They are, therefore, not being properly treated. If the child does improve that does not prove that they had a deficiency of the medication prescribed. Even children that do well on a stimulant drug are at risk for short-term and long-term side effects, and may need several dose adjustments as they continue to grow. Although I am not fond of drugs in general, I do realize that they have a role in patient treatment. I only wish to demonstrate that drugs are overused, overestimated in their efficacy, and underestimated in their safety profile. Several 'safe' drugs that have been studied with double-blind, randomized, placebo-controlled procedures, are later found to be dangerous and removed from the market. Many deaths have been attributed to *properly* prescribed drugs. Surely, many people have benefited from drugs, but is that the best and safest approach to all medical problems? Do we rely too much on drugs? What about for children with autism? Is drug therapy the answer? It is always rewarding to see a child with autism who has multiple health and behavioral challenges, be weaned off all their prescription drugs (under the supervision of a doctor) and given proper, safe, natural therapies and do well. There *is* a place for drugs. When a patient has a seizure disorder I use drug therapy to stop the seizures. For acute and <u>severe</u> recurrent pain syndromes including migraine headaches, I employ temporary drug therapy. Even in those cases, I still explore natural methods towards healing.

Pediatric neurologists are aware of seizure syndromes that are severe and refractory to drug therapy, but respond to natural interventions. A good example is vitamin B6 dependent seizures in infants. This conditions presents with severe, prolonged seizures controlled only by the administration of vitamin B6 (pyridoxine). Drugs do not work in this syndrome. Other conditions include vitamin and mineral deficiencies such as biotin and folinic acid. Refractory headaches can likewise be caused by specific mineral deficiencies like magnesium. With any medical condition, whether neurological or non-neurological, *incurable, refractory, intractable* cases may be ones whose proper treatment approach lies in a different paradigm. With biological interventions, it is best to focus on what the body needs. We should try to identify the underlying problem. If there are multiple problems, concentrate on the primary area of dysfunction, without ignoring the secondary factors, and work *with* the bodies natural healing mechanisms to mobilize *the doctor within.*

Mobilizing *the doctor within* simply means making sure that all the natural health laws are followed faithfully. How powerful and competent is *the doctor within* though? To answer this question we have to consider autoimmune disorders. Autoimmune disorders are an important category of medical illnesses. Up to 50 million Americans are thought to have some form of autoimmune disorder including conditions such as rheumatoid arthritis, multiple sclerosis, myasthenia gravis, and Hashimoto's thyroiditis. Interestingly, autism is now being viewed as a form of autoimmune disorder by many clinicians. Autoimmune disorders are crippling, disabling, and sometimes degenerative in nature. These conditions are examples of the powerful harm that can occur when *the doctor within,* in this case the immune system, attacks the wrong target, which is <u>one's own body</u>. An autoimmune disorder arises when the immune system starts attacking a person's own organs: the brain (in multiple sclerosis), the gut (in Crohn's disease), the joints (in rheumatoid arthritis), and the heart, kidneys and brain (in lupus). The havoc that is brought on by the attack is serious. The immune system is normally there to protect, defend, build up, repair, heal and restore the body. **The proof of its strength is the powerful damage it can cause when its force is unleashed against self.** Thomas Edison made a statement that we should all consider "the doctor of the future will give no medicines but will interest his patients in the care of the human frame, in diet, and in the cause and prevention of disease".

Psychosocial factors and the RESTORATION model

We live in such a fast paced, high expectation, individualistic society, that it is very easy to get overwhelmed and stressed. There are more and more individuals developing anxiety and mood disorders. Even young children are having 'nervous breakdowns'. In keeping with these problems, I see a subset of children referred to me for neurological problems such as refractory seizures, gait abnormalities, weakness, or chronic headaches that turn out to have severe emotional disturbances that account for what appears to be a neurological problem. In other words, seizures for instance, do not always have to be neurologic in origin. They can be psychogenic, the result of an emotional breakdown. An individual with non-epileptic seizures may not gain control of their seizures with seizure drugs. The individual does not have an incurable case of epilepsy. Simply, the wrong form of treatment is being implemented for this patient. This scenario is not uncommon. I had an adult patient whose seizures where so prolonged and unrelenting that the patient was about to be placed on a breathing machine (intubated) prior to being placed into a drug-induced coma to stop the seizures when it was discovered that the seizures were of psychogenic etiology. The patient revealed to the medical team that she was under a lot of stress and 'at the end of her rope'. Her stress was converted into an *apparent* seizure disorder. With appropriate counseling and support, this patient's seizures disappeared completely, **without seizure medicines**.

Many children with behavioral and academic difficulties of unclear etiology may have disorders that are largely psychogenic in origin. Others may have low self-esteem. These children could blossom in a supportive understanding environment where their underlying problem was understood. Many children get insufficient praise, which children need to thrive. Children need to believe in themselves. Their parents and teachers need to believe in them as well. And children need to *know* that their parents and teachers believe in them.

I took care of a child who had a lot of problems including a severe speech delay. This child's parents were told by other specialists that he would never talk because of the severity of his problems. He was almost 5 years old at that time. I saw him for several visits before he was lost to follow up. I saw him again after a couple of years and was pleasantly amazed to see that he was now speaking well and getting good grades in a mainstream classroom. I asked the family what made the difference in his language improvement. The answer was that he had moved to a new school where everyone believed in him and challenged him. He then blossomed! Interestingly, the child also became healthier. Previously, he had many illnesses. A happy, secure, appreciated child is more likely to be healthy compared to a child who is under a lot of stress with a poor self-esteem. Studies in the field of psychoneuroimmunology suggest that mental attitude and emotional status can influence the competence of the immune system, which in turn can alter neurological function. What this means is that a child with autism, who is receiving all of the appropriate therapies (behavioral, educational, and biomedical/nutritional) and that does not make the type of progress expected may be experiencing psychological disturbances that are holding him back.

Biology and psychology are interrelated. Psychosocial factors can have a significant impact on neurological, cognitive, and behavioral functioning. The reverse is also true. Biological, nutritional, metabolic, and immunologic disturbances can result in neuropsychiatric disturbances. This is because the brain chemicals that control and regulate our mood and sense of well-being (such as serotonin, the 'happy hormone') require proper nutritional intake for their synthesis. All of the hormones, neurotransmitters and other chemicals are in some way dependent on nutrients such as amino acids, trace elements, vitamins and water for their proper synthesis and metabolism. These are indispensable for optimal health.

You should be able to appreciate the various dimensions and factors involved in the treatment of complex neurobehavioral problems like autism. Restricting and limiting everything to the biological realm is inadequate. Psychosocial factors can be just as important in autism. Psychosocial factors are not just important for the patient, but for the family as well since they are ipso facto enmeshed in the child's illness. The child's illness extends to the parents. The child's anxiety may also be the parent's anxiety. The child's stress is the parent's stress. The learned helplessness and pessimism of the child may also become that of the parents'. This may in turn further aggravate the child's level of dysfunction. Proper restoration requires that positive changes be experienced not only by the affected child, but also by the parents and everyone else involved in the child's life.

Spiritual factors and the RESTORATION model

The spiritual portion of the **RESTORATION** model is the most crucial and unique. It forms the core from which the other aspects of the model derive. The spiritual aspects of the model are hope, faith, love, forgiveness, compassion and a belief in God. As human beings, we are not mere complex machines. If we were, medical science should by now be able to solve most of our medical dilemmas. In addition to a body, we have a mind and a spiritual dimension. The spiritual part of man may be hard for some people to fathom since it is intangible.

In the spiritual section of the Restoration model we explore the 'Why' questions. Why is a particular child born with a severe genetic disorder? Why is your child affected and not another? Why is one sibling affected and not the other? Why do some children seem to improve fast and not others? Why does God allow bad things to happen to good people? While science may be able to explain the 'how' of illness in many cases, it cannot answer the 'why'. When it comes to autism and other complex neuropsychiatric conditions, those who have failed all biomedical/ therapeutic interventions should consider looking into spiritual factors that may be the missing link.

The Science of Religion and the Religion of Science

Albert Einstein stated "Science without religion is lame, religion without science is blind", from Science, Philosophy and Religion: a Symposium, 1941.

Medical science deserves an 'A' when it comes to advances in medical technology and in acute/crisis-intervention situations, a 'B' when it comes to an understanding psychosomatic interactions since doctors are finally beginning to understand that mental conditions such as stress and emotional disturbances have an impact on virtually every aspect of physical health. When it comes to spiritual matters, medical science gets an 'F'. In conventional medicine, spirituality often plays a negligible role. It is interesting that the Diagnostic and Statistical Manual Mental Disorder fourth edition (DSM-IV) which is published by the American Psychiatric Association has started to acknowledge the role of religious or spiritual dysfunction in mental health. It has assigned a diagnostic code (V62.2) for *religious or spiritual problem* "when the focus of clinical attention is a religious or spiritual problem. Examples include distressing experiences that involve loss or questioning of faith, problems associated with conversion to a new faith, or questioning of spiritual values that may not necessarily be related to an organized church or religious institution". Although this is an embryonic step in the right direction, that is the *only* consideration that is given for religious problems among the numerous other conditions listed in the DSM-IV. Medicine has failed to assimilate the growing evidence that spirituality plays an important role in health. On the medical database of the National Library of Medicine there are thousands of articles dealing with spiritual and religious matters from prestigious medical centers throughout the country. One example was published in the Mayo Clinic Proceedings in 2001, from the Division of Internal Medicine, Department of Anesthesiology. This article reported that surveys suggest that "most patients have a spiritual life and regard their spiritual health and physical health as equally important. Furthermore, people may have greater spiritual needs during illness". The authors of the article reviewed other studies and have found that "most studies have shown that religious involvement and spirituality are associated with better health outcomes, including greater longevity, coping skills, and health-related quality of life (even during terminal illness) and less anxiety, depression, and suicide". Numerous articles have looked at the benefit of prayer with positive results.

When it comes to autism, there have been several shifts in the conceptual understanding of the disorder ranging from a psychiatric construct to psychodynamic and behavioral theories. Now there is a deeper understanding of the neurobiological and genetic factors. The last frontier to transcend beyond biomedicine and neuropsychiatry is the spiritual realm. In that sense, science and religion should compliment each other in that religious and scientific quests both have one main objective: finding truth.

A personal God

Laws must have a law giver. When you take into account that the human body conforms to a set of amazing principles, you are compelled to ask certain questions. Is this *intelligent* design really just a haphazard, spontaneous occurrence? Are the intricacies of human biology something that just evolved over time? I have chosen instead to believe that the intelligent design of the body, especially the brain, is no accident. I believe in the existence of a personal, loving God. I find great comfort in the knowledge that God has a name: Jehovah or Yahweh. I mention this because one of God's names is *Jehovah-Rophe* or "the Lord our Healer" (Exodus 15:26). I believe that all healing comes from God, the ultimate healer.

The Bible and Nutrition

In the Bible, Genesis 1:29, God told Adam and Eve that their diet should consist of "every seed bearing-plant on the face of all the earth and every tree that has fruit with seed in it." He said furthermore that "they will be yours for food". This statement has vital implications for us. First of all it entails believing in a Creator. One must consider that the Creator specifically designed our body to function properly, and has provided an operator's manual for us to maintain our bodies. In other words, by following a specific divine prescription, the body can function impeccably. So what does all of this have to do with autism? And, how does this pertain to spirituality? God has provided our bodies with special substances that He created to nourish the body and allow optimal development so that man could be at his best physically, psychologically, and spiritually. God knew that a body that was not well nourished would result in improper functioning of the brain, which is the organ of the mind and, hence the patient's spirituality would be compromised. Feeding the body properly by following God's initial dietary prescription, will result in biological health, and ultimately spiritual health. Therefore, it is important for us to take good care of our bodies. Based on the fact that man was initially given "every seed bearing-plant on the face of the earth and every tree that has fruit with seed in it" as food, it is logical to believe that God placed in nature everything the body needs to function properly. When considering children with autism, how closely does their diet adhere to God's original prescription for health? What would happen if these health laws *were* maintained in the lives of children with autism? What do fruits and herbs and vegetables contain that could restore children with autism to health?

It is interesting to note that fresh, raw, ripely-picked fruits and vegetables contain an impressive assortment of vitamins, minerals, antioxidants, fiber, water and perhaps thousands of phytochemicals that the body needs to function properly. It should not be a surprise from a nutritional standpoint that if children with ASD ate ALL of the required servings of raw fruits and vegetables daily, that they would function at a much higher level cognitively. The fruits and vegetables need to be harvested from rich soil, be ripely-picked, and pesticide-free. The sad reality is that most autistic kids are very picky eaters and have various oral, sensory, and texture limitations to foods. These children seem addicted to the common U.S. pediatric diet of junk food. The favorite meat source is chicken nuggets and the preferred 'vegetable' is French fries. These foods are given to the children not because they are nutritious, but because the children demand these foods. Many of these children who are receiving behavioral therapies receive candy or other refined sugars products as a reward for proper behavior.

Spiritual foods

God's natural laws also include *spiritual* foods such as faith, prayer, humility, patience, joy, and hope. As certainly as we need physical nourishment, we also need spiritual nourishment. There are also factors I call spiritual toxins such as hate, fear, pride, arrogance, dishonesty, that are more harmful than the deadliest physical toxins. These toxins also require a sort of detoxification, a spiritual one.

Prayer and Faith

Faith is one factor that is absolutely essential to health and healing. It is a belief that God has the power to heal. God's power starts where our strength ends. Faith, properly understood, has several components including: the *fear of the Lord*, abiding by His precepts, and asking for healing. Christ says "ask and it will be given to you". With faith one has to be persistent. Faith also entails implicit trust in God. It is fine to place your faith in doctors, therapies, and drugs, as long as you understand that all of these have limitations. Why not place your faith in God, who has the power to heal and restore. He created us, and, if necessary he can 'recreate' us.

Finally, with faith there is a time element. Not our time, but God's time. What would you do today if your child could suddenly talk? How would you behave if your child were restored to normal? God can make that happen, if He so desires, and if you are ready to give *Him* the praise, and if that experience will draw you closer to God. Prayer is an important avenue to God's throne. Prayer and faith are tools necessary for restoration to occur. When God is ready to heal, He is not interested in the timing of an injury, whether the damage is permanent or not, which specialists have already been seen, how soon interventions were started, what the mechanism of injury is, or what co-existing problems are present. He is only interested in the quality of your faith, and the sincerity of your prayer request. Some people lack humility, and are arrogant. It is impossible to please God if one lacks faith and humility.

Personal experience with prayer and faith

As a physician and specialist, I have never been afraid to call on Christ for help. There have been medical situations where I desperately needed God's help and He gave it to me in a miraculous way. There was a case of a patient who was admitted to the intensive care unit while I was on call. The patient went into an acute coma of undetermined etiology. I was contacted and ordered several tests. We were able to diagnosis a condition called acute disseminated encephalomyelitis where the brain and spine swell. This can be a serious condition. The patient developed increased pressure inside the skull because of the brain swelling to the point where a monitor was inserted through the skull. Unfortunately, the pressure kept rising until it was believed that was death imminent. The patient was in a deep coma, on a breathing machine with a catheter stuck through the skull. There was evidence of frequent seizures on the EEG. The prognosis was poor. One morning when I made my rounds, I felt like I needed to avoid the parents since I had no good news to offer them. Our best efforts were futile. As I wrote my note in the chart, the father approached me and desperately cried "if there is anything you can do to help my child, if you need to call on God's name, anything for my child". I must admit that I had not considered prayer up to that point, nor did the parent know about my religious beliefs. I asked "do you have faith in God's ability to heal." The answer was yes. With that, I held the parents' hands, asking God to heal and to restore the child, if it was His will. It was a short and simple prayer. I told the parents that it was now in God's hands.

Later, I was told that the pressure inside the skull was no longer increasing. It was coming down. There were no new medical interventions made to explain this occurrence. The intracranial pressure became normal. The patient awoke from the coma, and recovered quickly. The patient was transferred to a regular floor and eventually discharged. I saw the patient for follow up afterward, and was amazed to find that the patient had recovered completely with no residual neurological deficits. With tears in the eyes, the father told me that a miracle happened after we prayed in the ICU. There was complete restoration, not only of the sick and dying child, but for the entire family through the power of prayer and faith. In this particular situation, the medical institution was unable to save this patient. Everyone thought the child would die. But with divine intervention, the patient was completely cured. When I was praying for the child, another neurologist and some nurses in the room said I was crazy for praying and providing hope to this family. After the full recovery of this child, this neurologist stated "I guess your God does have the power to heal".

In an example like this, those that are skeptical might say that prayer had nothing to do with this child's recovery. Since disease 'just happens' you might also have cases of 'spontaneous remission' for no particular reason. Perhaps the girl was going to recover anyway, and the prayer was coincidental. I might consider such an argument, since even a serious illness can spontaneously resolve. However, how would one explain the father's smoking cessation? At the follow-up visit, the father related that after the prayer in the ICU a miracle occurred. The father, who was a chronic chain smoker for years, stopped smoking immediately after the prayer and has never picked up another cigarette, nor has he had the urge to do so. I did not know that he was a smoker before I prayed with him. My prayer was for the sick child. Along with the child's healing, however, the father was also restored. This is the *essence* of total restoration.

The above case has been a very important lesson for me personally since there are other situations where I would have wanted a similar miracle but did not experience it. I have come to the conclusion that God may not work a miracle when one is not needed. If there are available options that are ignored, the solution is to explore them.

When it comes to the condition of autism every child has the potential to recover. Every individual with autism can learn to communicate effectively. Isn't there something unique about autism that is admirable? This question is answered by the following poem written by Sondra William. She has autism.

They Say

I heard them talking about me, saying I am not like others.
I can dance and sing and play, I feel, and cry tears too.
I am more like you, than you think.

I heard them say that my silence reflects no emotion, no connection.
I cry many unseen tears, I laugh at life's blunders, although not in ways foreseen.
I connect like you, more than you think.

They say I am intellectually impaired and will never learn to reach my potential.
I know about words and explore the world in ways others rarely know.
I am smarter than you think.

The doctor says I will not be able to show affection or relate to my own family.
I gave them a smile from across the room, they didn't even notice.
I do know and feel love, more than you may think.

Some say my anger and the rages are animalistic.
I tried to communicate my fear the only way I know how, but no one was listening.
I get angry like you, for reasons like you, more than you think

The doctors say there is no hope, I am void of understanding.
I have dreams and think on them often, but due to my silence I can't share them.
Yes, I have dreams and goals, just like others, more than you think

Strangers say I am out of control and not human.
I have a body, mind and soul, just somewhat challenged.
I am human more than you think.

I heard them talking, saying oh, she has autism, a disability of no hope.
If they only know what is trapped inside me, I think.
They would say she's more like me, than what I use to think.

<u>Key points</u>

- Total restoration is possible for autism and other neuropsychiatric conditions.

- We have a powerful 'doctor within' and a well stocked natural 'internal pharmacy' that safely and competently takes care of all of our biological needs.

- Biological, psychological, social, and spiritual factors are important in restoring an individual to total health.

- Miracles may not be necessary when there are available options present.

- God is the all powerful, all loving Creator. He is the ultimate healer, so there is never any reason to lose hope!

CONCLUSION

In the case of autism and other complex neuropsychiatric conditions, there are a variety of effective treatment options that are available today that can allow children to overcome their difficulties. These children may require appropriate nutritional, behavioral, educational, and rehabilitative therapeutic interventions with some patience and optimism. Many children with autism and other neuropsychiatric conditions that struggle may do remarkably well later on in their development. Even children who appear delayed may do surprisingly well in the future. Who would have predicted that Albert Einstein, who did not talk until after the age of three and was a slow learner, would revolutionize the field of science? What about a boy who was thought to be severely mentally retarded and did not speak until he was almost four years old? This boy went on to revolutionize the way we all live with his 1,093 inventions. This boy was Thomas Edison. He had a mother who believed in him when no one else did. She was hopeful and optimistic. In reference to his mother he stated "…she was always so true and so sure of me and always made me feel I had someone to live for and must not disappoint". With hope, faith, trust in God, and proper management, people with autism and other neuropsychiatric disorders *are* able to be totally restored to health and wellness.

GLOSSARY OF IMPORTANT TERMINOLOGY

ABA (Applied Behavioral Analysis): A form of very intensive behavioral modification therapy. Behavior is broken down in units or discrete trials. Lovaas is the most popular form.

Agnosia: This is a term meaning 'lack of knowledge' applied to cognitive deficits in various areas. Pure word Agnosia (also called pure word deafness) found in conditions such as Landau-Kleffner syndrome is a condition where one cannot interpret the meaning of a particular word even if the sound of that word is heard. Generalized receptive language deficit can be thought of as a form of global agnosia.

AIT: This stands for auditory integration therapy and is a listening skill program. It re-educates the brain to perceive sound frequencies more accurately at unpredictable levels and intervals. There are many other listening skill programs like **Tomatis** (based on the relationship between hearing and phonation, therefore communication).

Alice in Wonderland syndrome: A syndrome where objects may appear unusually large or small.

Apraxia: An inability to perform a command although one may have the strength and general cognitive level of ability to do so. One form of apraxia is *verbal apraxia* where one is unable to figure out how to speak. Brain lesions may account for some cases of apraxia but neuroimaging may also be unrevealing in a lot of cases. In adults with sudden apraxia, stroke is always a consideration.

Asperger's Syndrome: A high functioning form of autism where an individual typically has normal to above normal intelligence. They may have narrowed interests and typically are very clumsy. There are significant social deficits present.

Aura: A sort of warning sign that indicates that a person is about to have a seizure. This can be an abnormal feeling in the gut or some strange behavior. Auras are usually very stereotypical and precede seizures by only a few minutes.

Casein: A protein found in dairy products. Some children with autism improve when this is completely removed from the diet. Intestinal symptoms and recurrent infections, as well as behavioral changes are common with casein sensitivity.

Casomorphine: A peptide caused from the improper breakdown of casein. It has opiate affects on the brain. It may cause an increased pain threshold, sensory processing abnormalities, aggressive behavior and 'brain fog' commonly encountered in children with autism.

Chelation: A process where a pharmacological agent is given orally, intravenously or trandermally to remove toxic heavy metals (e.g. mercury) stored in body tissues. Examples of chelating agents commonly used in autism include DMSA and DMPS.

Chelator: A special substance that has the ability to bind metal and cause its excretion from the body.

Coprographia: The writing of offensive language.

Coprolalia: The utterance of offensive words, swearing and bad language.

Copropraxia: The inappropriate use of obscene gestures.

Detoxification: The process of removing unwanted chemicals or toxins from the body

Echolalia: An involuntary repetition of another person's word.

Echopraxia: The involuntary imitation of another person's actions.

Emotional lability: Fancy medical term for mood swings.

Encephalopathy: A term used by neurologists to indicate brain disease from any number of causes. There are various types of encephalopathies including focal or generalized ones. *Static Encephalopathy* is a term used by pediatric neurologists to refer to non-progressive or static conditions such as cerebral palsy. [I strongly argue that autism and other autistic disorders should be classified as a *static encephalopathy*. This makes sense clinically and would avoid confusion as far as reimbursement from the insurance companies].

Epilepsy: A condition where cortical brain dysfunction causes someone to have recurrent seizures.

Gluten: A protein found in wheat, oat, and barley. Some children with autism improve when this is removed from the diet. Individuals with celiac disease also do not tolerate gluten. Intestinal and immune problems are common with gluten sensitivity.

Gut dysbiosis: An imbalance of gut flora (microorganism) that allows pathogens such as certain species of yeast or bacteria to overgrow while useful organisms such as probiotics (friendly bacteria) are deficient. This may result in secondary problems of behavior and neurological function.

Iatrogenic: A medical condition induced or caused by improper treatment. Examples include ailments caused by side effects of drugs. Some medical treatments may cause ailments that are far worse then the conditions that are being treated. This may also be the case in autism. In a broader sense, iatrogenic may refer to large scale practices that are detrimental.

Kanner's autism: Primary or classic autism. Usually it has an onset from early infancy and a more severe presentation.

Leaky gut syndrome: A condition of the gut whereby there is comprise of the barrier function of the intestines causing large molecules and toxins to pass through the gut wall. Gut dysfunction results in immune disturbances, food allergies, stress on the liver and further compromise of gastrointestinal function. This may contribute to autoimmune disturbances.

Locked-in syndrome: A neurological condition caused by a devastating stroke or trauma affecting particular parts of the brain. A victim is left without the ability to move, communicate, or respond though the mind is intact.

Macrocephaly: a larger than normal head size or circumference.

Metallothionein promotion therapy. A popular form of 'natural chelation' where zinc is given for several weeks along with vitamins to correct the functioning of a protein called metallothionein, which is involved in regulation of copper and zinc levels. After zinc loading, appropriate amino acids are supplemented. Metallothionein acts as a magnet for heavy metals and ultimately causes their excretion.

Microcephaly: a smaller than normal head size/circumference.

Mind-blindness: A theory pertaining to mental deficiencies in autism. According to this theory, individuals with autism are unable to perceive other people's thoughts or emotions.

Palilalia: An involuntary repetition of one's own words.

PDD: (Pervasive Developmental Disorder): A term introduced in the 1980s to describe a class of 5 apparently autistic conditions: autistic disorder, Rett syndrome, Childhood Disintegrative disorder, Asperger's syndrome and pervasive disorder not otherwise specified.

Pica: The habit of eating objects like dirt, flowers, leaves, or paper.

Placebo: An inert substance that when taken has a therapeutic effect.

Psychogenic: Pertaining to the mind or psychological factors. Psychogenic disturbances or disorders are ones that arise from an underlying emotional conflict perceived as extremely stressful. In these cases, there is a conversion of mental distress to bodily symptoms such as seizures (i.e. non-epileptic seizures), blindness or a number of other psychosomatic problems. Although psychogenic disturbances are *'non organic'* they are nonetheless real and require appropriate intervention.

Phenols: Chemical substances found in some foods including some fruits (citrus, apples, banana) and chocolate. Many individuals, who respond to the salicylate-free Feingold diet, may really have a problem tolerating phenols.

Rett's Syndrome: A neurodegenerative condition affecting females. They usually start with a normal head size that becomes smaller, with characteristic hand ringing and progressive development of autistic symptoms. Seizures are common. Any female child with autism, with a small head should be evaluated for Rett syndrome. The gene has been found for this disorder.

Regressive autism: A form of autism that is acquired. It occurs in a child who initially was progressing normally. Implications for this form of autism may be very different from the type that starts congenitally (from birth).

Self-stimulatory behavior or 'stimming': Abnormal repetitive movements such as hand flapping or rocking. Apart from motor forms, there can be visual or vocal forms as well. Among other factors, these behaviors are thought to serve a comforting function. These may increase in times of stress.

Specific carbohydrate diet: A dietary approach that is based on the idea that an increased carbohydrate load (specifically disaccharides and polysaccharides) is responsible for increased stress on the gastrointestinal tract. This stress is caused by abnormal yeast and bacteria that flourish by consuming these sugars. Therefore, eliminating those specific carbohydrates (but allowing simple monosaccharides like honey and fruit sugars in the diet) the gut to heal. Initially developed for conditions such as Crohn's disease and ulcerative colitis, many children with autism have tried this diet.

Sulfation Defect: A dysfunction of an enzyme called phenosulfotransferase which causes abnormalities in detoxification. A variety of allergy and headache symptoms are seen. Treatment with Epsom salt (magnesium sulfate) baths or cream may be useful.

Thimerosal: A preservative in vaccines, containing mercury.

APPENDICES

A) RECOMMENDED FOODS/BEVERAGES THAT SHOULD BE <u>AVOIDED</u> FOR BETTER HEALTH AND NEUROLOGICAL FUNCTIONING

- All dairy products (including milk, cheese, ice cream and yogurt)

  - Consider substituting with other forms such as soy or rice products. Soy, rice, or potato-based products exist for cheese, cream cheese, milk, ice cream, yogurt and other dairy products. Non-dairy products can be found in many regular stores.

- Caffeinated products (tea, coffee, chocolate, cola drinks)

- Processed meats (especially beef and pork)

- Fish contains omega 3 oils which are healthy. Be careful where you get fish due to possibility of heavy metal (e.g. mercury) toxicity.

- Drinks containing red dyes (e.g. Red dye #40)

  - Examples include: fruit punch

- Refined flour, sugar, bread

  - Consider whole wheat bread and brown rice

- Excessive sweets should be avoided

  - Consider natural sweeteners such as Stevia.

    - Avoid artificial sweeteners such as aspartame/NutraSweet

It is important to read labels. Avoid nitrates, MSG and other food chemicals with neurotoxic properties as much as possible.

Example of foods containing nitrates:

- Bologna, bacon, sausages, hotdogs, pepperoni, salami

- Commercial beef and hamburger meat

Example of foods containing MSG:

- Frozen foods

- Canned soups

- Processed meats

B) RECOMMENDED FOODS/BEVERAGES AND TYPES OF SUPPLEMENTS THAT SHOULD BE TAKEN FOR OPTIMAL HEALTH

- Plenty of fresh, raw, fruits and vegetables. Ideally, vine-ripened and pesticide-free. Some of the vegetables that contain the riches sources of potent phytochemicals and important substances such as glyconutrients include:

  - Broccoli

  - Carrots

  - Cauliflower

  - Cabbage

Since many children with autism and other conditions that involve oral defensiveness or texture problems may have great difficulty eating these very important foods. Consider juicing the vegetables and fruits. For best results, juice daily from the 5 color groups:

Green: Kiwi, broccoli (contain Indoles, Luteins)
Yellow/orange: Mango, carrots (contain carotenoids)
White: Bananas, cauliflower (contain allicin)
Red: Cranberries, tomatoes (contain lycopenes)
Blue/purple: Blueberries, eggplants (contain anthocyanins)

- Drink plenty of water. Drink the amount of water in ounces that is equal to approximately half of the body's weight in pounds.

- Multivitamins (dye-free, sugar-free). There are a variety of vitamin-like substances such as DMG/TMG that may be useful.

- Minerals.

- Essential fatty acids.

- Antioxidants.

- Probiotics.

- Glyconutrients.

In some cases where the diet is inadequate and deficiencies are present, amino acid supplementation may be necessary. Many children with multiple food allergies, gastrointestinal and immune problems may do very well with digestive enzymes. Extra fiber may be necessary in the diet. Consider working with a nutritionist or other professional knowledgeable in nutrition. Health food stores can be another source of information.

C) IMMUNIZATION CONCERNS: RECOMMENDATIONS

- Do not give more than 6 immunizations at one time.

- Make sure the child is in good health prior to receiving immunizations. If the child is ill, postpone the vaccines.

- Provide a regular daily multivitamin and give additional vitamins A and C prior to immunizations:

  Vitamin A < 2 years give 1250 IU
  2-5 years give 2500 IU
  5-10 years give 3750 IU
  > 10 years give 5000 IU

  Vitamin C Infants give 10 mg twice daily
  Toddlers give 300mg twice daily

  Give the vitamins the day prior, the day of, and the day after the immunizations are given.

- Consider giving the MMR vaccine individually.

- Be sure you vaccines are free of thimerosal.

Discuss any vaccination concerns with your physician.

D) STRATEGIES FOR DEALING WITH BEHAVIORAL AND COGNITIVE PROBLEMS SEEN IN CHILDREN WHITH AUTISM, ADHD AND RELATED CONDITIONS

- Keep the home organized, and establish a regular daily routine. Be consistent.

- Create a quiet non-distracting area for homework. Avoid over-stimulating situations when possible.

- Post rules, chores, and responsibilities.

- Make directions short, clear, and simple. Repeat instructions verbally and visually.

- Set small reachable goals.

- Give immediate frequent feedback.

- Reinforce positive behavior with toys, tokens, or privileges. Avoid negative comments.

- Plan ahead for new situations, transitions, or changes in routine to anticipate potential problem situations.

- Maintain consistency among parents and caregivers. Schedule regular free time or outlets for your child, and engage in pleasurable activities with your child regularly.

- Try keeping your child away from people or playmates who act aggressively.

- Do not roughhouse with an aggressive child. To do so may encourage aggressive behavior.

- Always try to distinguish between non-compliance (won't) and inability (can't).

- Enhance the child's self-esteem by focusing on the child's strength. Find activities at which your child can succeed. Refrain from all forms of verbal abuse.

E) RECOMMENDATIONS FOR SLEEP DISTURBANCES

Sleep disturbances can result from a variety of underlying problems which should be treated when present. Examples include:

- Primary sleep disturbance (e.g. insomnia, sleep apnea)

- Pain disorders

- Depression

- Chronic anxiety

- Systemic illness

- Nocturnal seizures

Proper nutrition and exercise are important in helping with good quality sleep. Avoid caffeine. Avoid noise. Avoid overly stimulating activities right before going to bed. There should not be a noisy environment in the bedroom.

Consider using a natural sleep supplement. Examples include:

- Melatonin (0.5-5mg. Liquid, Lozenges, Sublingual tablets, tablet forms available)

- GABA (150 mg capsules. Take 1-8 capsules or 150-1200 mg)

- Taurine (325 mg capsules. Take 1-4 capsules or 325-1300mg per day)

- Valerian (400-900mg. Take up to 2 hours before bedtime).

There are various other products that contain mixtures of melatonin, GABA, threonine, glycine, and valerian. Always consider a medical evaluation if proper sleep cannot be obtained since sleep is vital to health and healing.

F) SUBTLE SIGNS OF SEIZURES

- Staring spells, with altered responsiveness

- Dazed behavior

- Confusion

- Brief periods of unresponsiveness

- Facial, eyelid, or lip twitching usually with some alteration in consciousness as opposed to a motor tic where ther should be no change in consciousness or awareness.

- Spontaneous eye rolling. This can also be seen in some tic disorders.

- *Unprovoked* outbursts with altered consciousness.

- Spontaneous mirthless, mechanical laughter. Children with autism often have giggling spells for other reasons which include toxic states, nutritional imbalance, or an infectious source like yeast.

- Unexplained drowsiness.

- Intermittent clumsiness or gait disturbance.

Always try to assess the level of awareness and responsiveness during a suspected seizure. All suspected cases of seizures require medical evaluation.

G) POTENTIAL TRIGGERS FOR HEADACHES AND SEIZURES

- Fever

- Infection

- Physical or emotional Stress

- Sleep depravation and excessive fatigue

- Environmental Factors

  - Bright or flickering light, such as video games (these are called photic stimulation)

  - Weather changes

- Food and chemicals

  - Nitrates

  - MSG

There is an important subset of children who have both headaches and seizures. Sometimes an individual may have a headache that precedes, occurs during, or follows certain types of seizures. Although some of the above triggers may play a greater role in either headaches or seizures, they all can directly or indirectly affect both conditions and should thus be avoided. If headaches or seizures are present, always keep a diary. The diary should include the following information:

- Date/Time

- Severity (in case of headache on a scale of 1-10)

- Description (in case of seizures)

- Duration

- Precipitating factors

  - Food/drink consumed within the past 4 hours (in the case of headaches).

H) POSSIBLE SYMPTOMS OF DETOXIFICATON

Detoxification is the process the body uses to get rid of accumulated toxins in the body. Some individuals, who alter their lifestyle in a positive manner, may at times experience detoxification symptoms, especially in the beginning of a treatment. Although the process of detoxification can cause symptoms, this should not be a reason to quit removing toxins from your body.

Cause of detoxification symptoms

- Prior to leaving the body, toxins are expelled from tissues and circulate in the bloodstream.

- Toxins exit the body via several systems (e.g. the skin) which can cause temporary symptoms in those areas.

- During detoxification, the body is able to absorb things better, including harmful food substances (e.g. caffeine, refined sugar) that may cause worse than usual symptoms.

- Sometimes people give up meats during detoxification, and discover that they are more fatigued than usual. This is because the protein in meat is stimulating, and once it is removed from the diet the person becomes more tired. This is a temporary effect of detoxification and will resolve.

The duration and severity of detoxification symptoms may vary. In some cases, instead of being linear, the symptoms can be cyclical.

Examples of Detoxification Symptoms

- Fatigue

- Clogged Skin

- Skin Rash

- Fever

- Cough

- Cold Symptoms

- Gas

- Stomachache

- Diarrhea

- Constipation

- Headache

- Moodiness

- Irritability

REFERENCES

ALTERNATIVE THERAPIES

Commonly used herbal medicines in the United States: a review. S. Bent, MD ad R. Ko, PharmD, PhD. American Journal of Medicine. Volume 116, Number 7, April 1, 2004.
Herbal Cures for Common Ailments. Jim O'Brien. Globe Digests. 1997.
The Antioxidant Miracle. Lester Packer, PhD & Carol Colman. 1999.
Treatment choice is ultimately the patient's. M. Fleming, MD. American Medical News. Page 19, October 4, 2004.

GLUTEN/CASEIN-FREE DIET

Adv. Biochem. Psychopharmacol. 28: 27-643.
Autism 1999; 3:45-65.
Brain Dysfunction, 3 (1990): 308-19.
Brain Research 412 (1987) p. 68-72.
Dev Brain Dysfunct 7 (1994) p. 71-85.
Journal of Applied Nutrition 42 no. 1 (1990) 1-11.
Oski, Frank A. (1992) Don't Drink Your Milk! New Frightening Medical Facts About The Worlds Most Overrated Nutrient, 9th Edition. Teach Services: Burshton, NY.
Panksepp J Trends in Neurosciences 2 (1979) p. 174-177.

AUTISM AND BEHAVIOR

Journal of Consulting and Clinical Psychology. 1987, Vol. 55, No 1.3-9.
Advocate 1994. Interview with Ivar Lovaas.

AUTISM EPIDEMIC

Blaxil MF—Public Health Rep-01-NOV-2004; 119 (6): 536-51.

CDC, April 2000. "Prevalence of Autism in Brick Township, New Jersey, 1998: Community Report".

Croen LA—J Autism and Developmental Disorders 01—June-2002; 32 (3):217-24.

Disabilities Education Act, Table, AA11. pp 6-21.

Fombonne E—J Autism Dev Disord-01-AUG-2003; 33(4):365-82.

Lancet 1997; 350:1761-6.

Merrick J—Int J Adolesc Med Health—01—Jan—2004; 16 (1):75-8.

22nd Annual Report to Congress on the Implementation of the individuals with Pediatrics Vol. 107 No. 2 February 2001, pp. 411-412.

U.S. News & World Report, June 19, 2000 p.47.

Yeargin-Allsopp M-JAMA—1—Jan-2003; 289 (1): 49-55.

B6 AND MAGNESIUM

Ann NY Acad Sci 1990; 585: 250-60.

Biol Psychiatry 1991 May 1; 29 (9) 931-41.

Dev Med Child Neurol 1989 Dec; 31 (6): 721-7.

J. Autism Dev Disord 1995 Oct; 25 (5): 481-93.

J. Autism Dev Disord 1998 Dec; 28 (6) 581-2.

J. Child Neurol 1988; 3 Suppl: S68-72.

AUTISM AND SEIZURES

Advances in Neurology 1986; 501-12.

Arch Neurol 1988; 45:666-668.

Epilepsia, 1989, 30, 90-93 (improvement of seizures with DMG).

J AM Acad Child Psychiatry 1990:29z; 127-129.

New England Journal of Medicine 1982, 307, 1081-1082 (improvement of seizures with DMG).

Pediatrics 1999 Sep; 104 # 405-18 *82% of children with ASD have clinically relevant abnormality on EEG (MEG).*

GUT PROBLEMS (DYSBIOSIS) IN AUTISM

Acta Paediatr 1998 Aug; 87 (8) 836-4.

Clin Sci (Colch) 2000 Aug; 99 (2): 93-1-4.

Dig Dis Sci. 2000 Apr; 45(4)723-9.

Gut 2002 May; 50 Suppl 3: III60-III54.
J. Assoc Acad Minor Phys. 1998; 9 (1):9-15.
J. Child Neurol. 2000 Jul: 15(7):429-35.
J. Pediatr 1999 Nove; 135 (5):559-63.
Lancet. 1998 Feb 28; 351 (9103): 637-41.
Lancet. 2000 Aug 26; 356 (9231).
Mol Psychiatry 2000;7 (4):375-82.
Pediatr. 2001 Mar; 138(3): 366-72.
Proc Natl Acad Sci USA 1999 Oct 12;96 (21) 12012-7.
Toxicol Ind Health 1998 Jul-Aug; 14 (4) 553-63.

DETOXIFICATION PROBLEMS

J. Nutri Enviro Med 2000; 10 (1):25-32.
J. Orthomolec. Med., 8(4) 198-200.
Toxicology 1996; 111:43-65.

FOOD SENSITIVITIES/ADDITIVES

Annals of Allergy 1994, 72(5) 462-468.
Annals of Allergy 1994, 73 (3) 215-19.
J. Orthomolec 1993. Med., 8 (4).
Panminerva Med 1995 Sep; 37(3): 137-41.
Scand J Educaional Res 1995; 39: 223-36.

THIMEROSAL AND AUTISM

Amy Holmes, Mark Blaxill Reduced Levels of Mercury in and Body Haley International Journal of Toxicology, 22:277-285, 2003. First Baby Haircuts.
Molecular Psychiatry 2004, 1-13. Neurotoxic Effects of Postnatal Thimerosal are Mouse Strain Dependent.

AUTOIMMUNITY AND AUTISM

Annals of Neurology. Neuroglial Activation and Neuroinflammation in the Brain of Patients with autism. Online publication. November 15, 2004.
Pediatrics 01-NOV-2003; 112 (5): E420 Increased prevalence of familial autoimmunity with pervasive developmental disorders.

MISC

Kanner L. Autistic disturbances of affective contact. Nerv. Child 2:217-50. 1943

Ohnishi et al. Brain vol. 123, No 9, 1938—1844. Abnormal regional cerebral blood flow in childhood autism.

Mueller PS et al. Religious involvement, spirituality, and medicine: implications for clinical practice. Mayo Clin Proc. 2001 Dec: 76 (12):1225-35

Megson, Mary. Is autism a G-alpha protein defect reversible with natural vitamin A? Abstract. (See omega-research.com).

BOOKS:

1. A Guide to Scientific Nutrition for Autism and Related Conditions. By Kirkman Laboratories.

2. Autism. Explaining the Enigma. By Uta Frith

3. Autism. The Facts. By Dr. Simon Baron-Cohen and Dr. Patrick Bolton

4. Behavioral Intervention for Young Children with Autism. By Catherine Maurice.

5. Beyond the Wall. Personal Experiences with Autism and Asperger Syndrome. By Stephen Shore.

6. Biological Treatments for Autism and PDD. By William Shaw, Ph.D.

7. Children with Starving Brains: A Medical Treatment Guide for Autism Spectrum Disorder. By Jacquelyn McCandless, MD.

8. Conquering Autism. Reclaiming Your Child Through Natural Therapies. By Stephen Edelson, MD

9. Diagnostic and Statistical Manual of Mental Disorders Fourth edition (DSM-IV). Published by the American Psychiatric Association

10. Enzymes for Autism and other Neurological Conditions. The Practical Guide for Digestive Enzymes and Better Behavior. By Karen DeFelice

11. Facing Autism: Giving Parents Reasons for Hope and Guidance for Help. By Lyn M. Hamilton.

12. How to Survive on a Toxic Planet. By Dr. Steve Nugent

13. Milk the Deadly Poison. By Robert Cohen

14. Mind-blindness. An Essay on Autism and Theory of Mind. By Simon Baron-Cohen

15. Oski, Frank A. (1992) Don't Drink Your Milk! New Frightening Medical Facts about the Worlds Most Overrated Nutrient, 9th Edition. Teach Services: Burshton, NY.

16. Special Diets for Special Kids. By Lisa Lewis, Ph.D.

17. Textbook of Pediatric Neuropsychiatry. By Edward Coffey, M.D. and Roger Brumback, M.D.

18. The Out of Sync Child. By Carol Kranowitz.

19. Thinking in Pictures: And Other Reports From My Life with Autism. By Temple Grandin.

20. Unraveling the Mystery of Autism and Pervasive Developmental Disorder: A Mother's Story of Research and Recovery. By Karyn Seroussi.

21. What Your Doctor May Not Tell you About Children's Vaccinations. By Stephanie Cave, M.D., F.A.A.F.P.

WEBSITES:

www.autism.com/ari
www.vaporia.com/autism/
www.gnd.org
www.gfcfdiet.org
www.AutismNDI.com

ABOUT THE AUTHOR

Dr. Jean-Ronel Corbier is a board certified pediatric neurologist who specializes in the treatment of autism. His background is unique in that he grew up in several different countries. He lived in Africa with his parents as missionaries for 7 years. This exposure greatly broadened his perspective on life. He went to medical school at Michigan State University College of Human Medicine. He completed his neurology training at the University of Cincinnati and Children's Hospital of Cincinnati. He has also completed neurology electives at Johns Hopkins, the Mayo Clinic and the University of Michigan. While in medical school, he enrolled concurrently in a graduate program in Health and Humanities. This gave him the opportunity to work on several projects with alternative health professionals. Dr. Jean-Ronel Corbier has been investigating the role of nutrition in the treatment of neurological disorders, and might be thought of as a pediatric nutritional neurologist. This background along with Dr. Corbier's strong Christian faith, gives him a broad and unique perspective on the complex disorder of autism. Dr. Jean-Ronel Corbier currently practices pediatric neurology in Montgomery, Alabama. His wife is a pediatrician, and they have one son.

0-595-34892-0